TEENAGE NUTRITION AND PHYSIQUE

TEENAGE NUTRITION
AND PHYSIQUE

By

RUTH L. HUENEMANN, D.Sc.
Professor of Public Health Nutrition

MARY C. HAMPTON, M.S.
Associate Specialist

ALBERT R. BEHNKE, M.D.
U.S.N. Ret., Lecturer

LEONA R. SHAPIRO, M.S.
Lecturer

and

BARBARA W. MITCHELL, M.S.
Statistician

Nutrition Program
School of Public Health
University of California
Berkeley, California

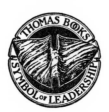

CHARLES C THOMAS · PUBLISHER
Springfield · Illinois · U.S.A.

Published and Distributed Throughout the World by
CHARLES C THOMAS · PUBLISHER
Bannerstone House
301-327 East Lawrence Avenue, Springfield, Illinois, U.S.A.

© 1974, by CHARLES C THOMAS · PUBLISHER
ISBN 0-398-03135-5
Library of Congress Catalog Card Number: 74 1013

*With THOMAS BOOKS careful attention is given to all details of manufacturing
and design. It is the Publisher's desire to present books that are satisfactory as to
their physical qualities and artistic possibilities and appropriate for their particular
use. THOMAS BOOKS will be true to those laws of quality that assure a good
name and good will.*

Printed in the United States of America
K-8

Library of Congress Cataloging in Publication Data
Main entry under title:

Teenage nutrition and physique.

Bibliography: p.
1. Youth—Health and hygiene. 2. Youth—Nutrition.
3. Corpulence. I. Huenemann, Ruth L
[DNLM: 1. Adolescent psychology. 2. Body composi-
tion—In adolescence. 3. Nutrition—In adolescence.
QU145 T258 1974]
RJ140.T43   613.7′04′3   74–1013
ISBN 0-398-03135-5

PREFACE

THIS REPORT DEALS with body size, composition and conformation of a teenage population and associated factors. It describes the purpose, methods and findings of a four-year longitudinal and cross-sectional study conducted in Berkeley, California, during the years 1961 to 1965. Subjects numbered roughly 1,000 teenagers each year, studied at successive grade levels from nine through twelve. Body composition and conformation were assessed annually for the entire sample, as were subjects' views regarding body size and shape, food and activity. Definitive studies of body composition, food intake, and activity were conducted with a subsample of approximately 200 subjects.

The study was prompted by current public health concern with obesity and lack of physical fitness as conditions possibly contributing toward cardiovascular disease. Findings regarding prevalence of obesity and factors associated with it will doubtless be of interest to physicians, nurses, nutritionists, physical education and classroom teachers, dietitians, home economists, school lunch personnel, and others. The successive assessments of gross body composition, size and shape of present-day teenagers will augment the relatively small amount of data on this aspect of human development. The detailed tables of body measurements might well interest the garment manufacturer. Information about food practices, eating frequency, and teenage views on food and eating will probably capture the attention not only of the health professional, but also of food scientists and the food industry. The social scientist may find the case histories interesting as a reflection of teenage living.

Physicians, physiologists, anthropometrists, physical education experts and others will be interested in a companion volume

v

by Albert R. Behnke and Jack H. Wilmore entitled, "Evaluation and Regulation of Body Build and Composition," * which synthesizes and interprets data from the study with data from other studies.

The investigators hope that their findings will prove to be especially helpful to those professional people planning programs designed to maintain the health of teenagers through improved nutrition and increased physical activity, both of which are related to control of obesity.

* New York, Academic Press, 1972.

ACKNOWLEDGMENTS

THE STUDY WAS SUPPORTED by a grant from the National Institute of Child Health and Human Development, National Institutes of Health, Public Health Service, U.S. Department of Health, Education, and Welfare. Additional assistance was supplied by a General Research Support Grant for School of Public Health statistical services and the services of Feleni Schulz Little, editor. Statistical consultant was Alvin D. Wiggins, Ph.D., and programming was done by William Quinn, Christina Gibson, and Michael Vendeman. Elizabeth Hayes also assisted with the data processing. Additional data analyses were supplied by the Survey Research Center of the University of California, Berkeley.

The Nutrition Foundation supplied financial support for the preparation and printing of this monograph.

We are grateful for the assistance supplied by our interviewing nutritionists, Ann Burroughs, Margaret Ostrom, Dorothy Pearson, Claudine Reed, and June Whitaker.

Rita Bonge and Lin Heald deserve special thanks for the long hours spent at the typewriter in preparing the manuscript and Lynne Ramsey for her assistance with typing and clerical work.

The generous and unfailing cooperation of the Berkeley City Department of Public Health and the Berkeley Unified School District is gratefully acknowledged.

The project was possible only with the cheerful cooperation of the many teenagers who were the subjects.

Ruth L. Huenemann
Mary C. Hampton
Albert R. Behnke
Leona R. Shapiro
Barbara W. Mitchell

CONTENTS

Preface v

Acknowledgments vii

Chapter

    1. PURPOSE 3

    2. THE SAMPLE AND PROCEDURE 6

    3. ANTHROPOMETRIC FINDINGS 10

    4. CALORIC AND NUTRIENT INTAKES AND EATING
       PRACTICES 46

    5. RECORDED ACTIVITIES AND ATTITUDES TOWARD
       ACTIVITIES 81

    6. SCHOOL PERFORMANCE 96

    7. TEENAGERS' ATTITUDES 127

    8. IMPLICATIONS 147

Bibliography 155

Appendices 159

TEENAGE NUTRITION AND PHYSIQUE

CHAPTER 1

PURPOSE

CURRENT CONCERN with obesity, lack of physical fitness, diabetes and cardiovascular disease has resulted in renewed interest in the matter of body composition and conformation. This monograph describes a four-year longitudinal and cross-sectional study of body size, shape, and composition of approximately 1,000 teenagers in Berkeley, California. The association of food and activity with body composition and conformation was investigated in a subsample of about 200. Specifically, the aims of the study were:

1. to determine by annual anthropometric measurements over a four-year period the body size, conformation, growth, and development of approximately 1,000 teenage boys and girls of various racial backgrounds in one city in Western United States;
2. to obtain a measure of the food intake and physical activity of these teenagers and to determine possible meaningful associations that might exist between these and body composition, body conformation, sex, age, race, and socioeconomic status;
3. to utilize the body measurement data, along with those from other studies of teenagers and other age groups, to substantiate a body of principles regarding body composition, conformation, and growth;
4. to determine the prevalence of obesity, the time of onset, and, if possible, the relative effects of food intake and physical activity on its occurrence. We hoped that by such systematic study of the development of obesity we might discover ways of identifying the potentially obese, so that

high-risk groups might be led into obesity-prevention programs;

5. to determine associations between body measurements and performance as indicated by standardized physical performance tests, school attendance, school grades;

6. to test the feasibility of the methods employed for use in a public school setting;

7. to validate by independent methods applied to a subsample the accuracy of the method employed to determine gross body composition;

8. to learn something of teenagers' own views on body size and build, physical activity, and food intake; and to determine whether or not these stated views appear to be associated with body composition.

In general, the purpose of this descriptive study was to obtain data useful for planning programs in public health nutrition.

The major areas of this study have been previously investigated and are currently under study by others. Purposes, methods, and subjects have differed from those of this study, as have time and place. Assessment of teenage body composition, growth, and nutrition constituted part of the longitudinal studies of Garn and Haskel (1959), Reynolds (1946), and others of the Fels Research Institute; those of Falkner (1958), Tanner (1955), and others at the Child Development Unit of the University of London; of Washburn (1957) and staff of the Denver Child Research Council. The older work of Stuart and associates (1947), is a classic in the field. A multifaceted growth study of California boys and girls was carried out several decades ago by Jones (1938), Pryor (1936), Tuddenham and Snyder (1954), and others.

The Agricultural Experiment Stations conducted extensive cross-sectional studies of nutritional status and food intake of teenagers throughout the United States during the period of 1947 to 1958. They included biochemical assessment of nutritional status, height, weight, and in some instances assessment of body fat by skinfold calipers. Morgan (1959) summarized those studies. Johnson (1956), Stefanik (1959), and Bullen and colleagues (1963), studied the role of activity, food, psychological factors, and body composition of family members in relation to obesity in teenagers. Eppright and coworkers (1955) investigated the dietary intakes of Iowa girls in relation to obesity and leanness. Hinton (1962) studied the physiological, psychological, and sociological factors that might be related to eating behavior and selection of an adequate diet. Further reference to the above and other studies will be made in subsequent chapters wherever comparisons with them are in order.

Radical changes have occurred in the American way of life during the past decade—changes which may well reflect in the body composition, food practices, activities, and preferences of teenagers. Therefore, studies made even ten years ago may no longer characterize the present situation. California youth, reputed to live an outdoor type of life, may differ from their contemporaries in other parts of the country. The sample for this study makes interracial comparisons possible. All of these variations from studies done elsewhere or in previous decades, in addition to local public health interest in teenagers, prompted our present investigation and constitute our justification for this report.

CHAPTER 2

THE SAMPLE AND PROCEDURE

AN EXPEDIENT WAY of reaching a teenage population for repeated study seemed to be to follow one entire grade of the city's public school population through its remaining high school years. Accordingly, the ninth grade of the year 1961 was chosen at that time as the population for study. This was an interracial group, with roughly one-third of the class Negro, one-tenth Oriental, and the remainder Caucasian in ethnic origin (Table 2-I). We made the ethnic classification by visual observation. Those whose race was not obvious by observation were classified as "unknown." Since in the Berkeley school system progression from one grade to the next is regular, children of one grade level were within a few months of the same age. Mean ages of our subjects for the four years were 14.5, 15.3, 16.3 and 17.3 years. As ninth graders they were attending three separate junior high schools. For the remaining three years of the study they were in the city's only senior high school. The total number examined each year will be referred to as the total sample, and the subjects for whom we have data for all four years will be referred to as the longitudinal sample.

For more definitive tests, we chose a subsample of about 200 students to include comparable numbers of those with the lowest, the highest, and the medium range of body fat as determined anthropometrically during the preceding school year. This group will be referred to as the subsample and those for whom four complete weeks of data were obtained, the longitudinal subsample.

The sample consisted of all students that could be contacted in their physical education classes where they were measured in each grade each year. As can be seen in Table 2-I, the number in

TABLE 2–I

TOTAL SUBJECTS FOR FOUR YEARS

Mean Age (Years)	Year 1 14.5		Year 2 15.3		Year 3 16.3		Year 4 17.3		Longi- tudinal Sample
TOTAL MEASURED									
Boys									
Caucasian	267		258		250		224		121
Negro	137		152		168		140		74
Oriental	44		36		37		35		27
Unknown	10		8		11		4		5
Total	458	458	454	454	466	466	403	403	227	227
Girls									
Caucasian	316		268		245		245		160
Negro	147		142		139		117		59
Oriental	42		34		36		37		29
Unknown	14		8		3		5		6
Total	519	519	452	452	423	423	404	404	254	254
		977		906		889		807		481
TOTAL QUESTIONNAIRES									
Boys									
Caucasian	240		235		241		249		113
Negro	113		144		139		145		59
Oriental	43		36		35		37		29
Unknown	69		36		11		29		5
Total	465	465	451	451	426	426	460	460	206	206
Girls									
Caucasian	303		261		244		231		156
Negro	130		147		142		111		63
Oriental	40		38		36		33		30
Unknown	46		37		5		4		1
Total	519	519	483	483	427	427	379	379	250	250
		984		934		853		839		456
MEASUREMENT PLUS QUESTIONNAIRES									
Boys									
Caucasian	240		229		239		216		
Negro	113		130		138		125		
Oriental	43		32		35		35		
Unknown	6		5		11		4		
	402	402	396	396	423	423	380	380	
Girls									
Caucasian	303		250		244		229		
Negro	130		134		136		102		
Oriental	40		34		36		34		
Unknown	11		7		4		4		
	484	484	425	425	421	421	369	369	
		886		821		844		749		

the longitudinal sample was considerably smaller than the total sample.

Each year, after collecting the data, we classified our sample in two ways, by race and by amount of body fat. We divided our sample arbitrarily into five groups for each sex by a frequency distribution of percent of body fat as determined by body envelope. According to the method of Behnke (1961, 1963a, 1963b, 1972), we called the ten percent with the least amount of body fat "lean," the next fifteen percent "somewhat lean," the middle fifty percent "average," the next fifteen percent "somewhat obese" and the ten percent with the largest amount of body fat we called "obese." (These classifications were also applied in other phases of this study to questionnaire data, dietary intake data, activity record data, and school performance data.)

Questionnaire data were collected each year, also. Two questionnaires were designed to yield information regarding teenagers' preferences, views, and knowledge about food and eating, body conformation, and activity. The first, given to subjects in the ninth grade, dealt primarily with their views on food and activity. The second, used in the tenth grade, focused on body composition and conformation and included views on food and activity only in relation to body structure. Because particularly meaningful information was gained from three questions from the first questionnaire given to the ninth grade, we asked the same questions in the eleventh grade for comparison. For the same reason, we gave the second questionnaire and selected questions from the first again in the twelfth grade.

Questionnaires were distributed to students to be answered during regular physical education class periods under the supervision of teachers or project personnel.

For reporting some of the data, the sample was also classified by socioeconomic status. Socioeconomic levels were based on 1960 census data (U.S. Census of Population, 1960). This table gives family income in $999-increments and the number and percent of all Berkeley families in each increment. Using these data the one-third and two-thirds family income levels were determined, and lower-third, middle-third, and upper-third family income ranges developed.

lower third: less than $5,110
middle third: $5,111 to $8,586
upper third: $8,587 and above

Median family income for each of the 29 Berkeley census tracts was also available from 1960 census data. Students were put into a socioeconomic level based on the median family income of the census tract in which they lived.

We asked our subsample subjects to keep a diary each day for seven consecutive days to include what was eaten, the amount, method of preparation, and time of day it was consumed, as well as to record time spent in various activities. We obtained four of these weekly diaries: one each from the summer of 1963, the spring of 1964, the summer of 1964, and the spring of 1965. While keeping the diaries, the subjects were asked to visit our offices each day (except Sunday) so that we might check their previous day's diary.

Interviewers were home economists or nutritionists who were instructed to maintain an interested, but nonjudgmental, attitude toward any recorded behavior. Each interviewer was responsible for coding the dietary and activity data obtained from each of her interviewees for computer processing (U.S. Dept. of Health, Education and Welfare, 1964).

We appealed to the subjects in the subsample to help us as scientists. We explained that it was important for us to obtain scientifically accurate information about what they ate and did; and that they were the only people who could provide this information. Therefore, they were scientists collecting data for us. The appendix contains some of the forms and letters we distributed to the subsample subjects.

The entire project was made possible by the close cooperation of three agencies: The Berkeley Unified School District; The School of Public Health, University of California; and The City of Berkeley Department of Public Health.

CHAPTER 3

ANTHROPOMETRIC FINDINGS*

S PECIFIC OBJECTIVES for the anthropometric phase of this study
were to determine the prevalence of obesity and the time of
its onset in our subjects; to identify the obese and any factors
that might be related to their obesity; to discover ways of identifying the potentially obese so that high-risk groups or individuals might be led into obesity prevention programs; to investigate any racial differences in body composition or conformation
in order to determine if the same standards should be applied to
all ethnic groups; to study the growth of our subjects in their
teen years; to test the Behnke (1961, 1963a, 1963b, 1972) anthropometric method of assessing body build and composition
with respect to its use in a public school; to check the Behnke
(1961, 1963a, 1963b, 1972) method by applying other methods
to selected subsamples.

Methods of Assessing Body Composition

All methods of assessing body composition *in vivo* are indi-
rect, and all have limiting features. Some more precise methods
of measuring body composition, such as determining density by
underwater weighing (Behnke, 1942) or helium dilution (Siri,
1956) and counting of radioactive potassium (Forbes, Gallup
and Hursh, 1961), are limited by time and equipment required.
Height and weight data applied to a standard such as the Wetzel
Grid (Wetzel, 1941) have the obvious drawback of defining only
a degree of overweight or underweight compared with average
values, and identify no other physical feature of the subject. Ob-
servational ratings of obesity can be done quickly and are more

* A portion of this chapter appeared originally in the *American Journal of Clin-
cal Nutrition, 19:*422, December, 1966, to which we are indebted for its use.

descriptive than height and weight data alone but have the disadvantage of being subjective.* Measurements of skinfolds (Keys and Brozek, 1953), give values for the quantities of subcutaneous fat and are useful for comparison. Young and associates (1961) found skinfold thickness to be a fairly reliable indicator of relative fatness. However, we thought it might be difficult to get reproducible results because we required several technicians to obtain data from a large sample.

The Behnke (1961, 1963a, 1963b, 1972) anthropometric method seemed the most suitable for use in the public school setting. A trained technician could measure the height, weight, circumferences, and diameters of one student in five to ten minutes. Since our study was part of the school program, the Behnke method provided a further advantage to the students and teachers because it permitted us to prepare somatograms for the subjects. (See Figure 3–1.) We found that the somatograms † were of great value in maintaining the interest of our subjects in the study.

* Medical examinations were done on some of our subjects by an independent research group (The California Joint Study of Student Health Problems and School Performance). Of the subjects examined, eight boys and three girls were obese by our standards. The examining physicians, however, mentioned overweight as a health problem for only two boys.
* The percent of age deviation from the k values (based on average body configuration) for the body measurements gives a diagramatic representation of that individual's deviation from the norm.

Calculation of percent deviation from subject's own average for each measurement in order to draw profile or somatogram is shown:

$$\text{Percent deviation} = \frac{\text{Measurement's \% of Total Measurements} - \text{k value}}{\text{k value}}$$

k Values:

Measurement	Females	Males
Shoulder	17.33	18.47
Chest	14.83	15.30
Abdomen	12.90	13.53
Buttocks	16.93	15.57
Thigh	10.03	9.13
Biceps	4.80	5.13
Forearm	4.33	4.47
Wrist	2.73	2.73
Knee	6.27	6.10
Calf	6.13	5.97
Ankle	3.70	3.60
Total	99.98	100.00

Note: Height is always used in decimeters.

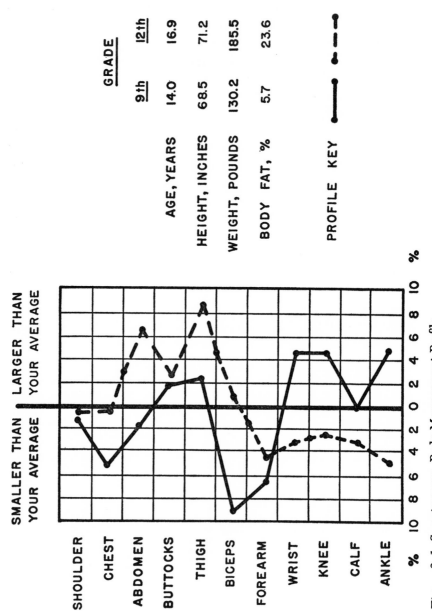

Figure 3–1. Somatograms. Body Measurement Profile.

All measurements of subjects were done or supervised by A. R. Behnke. Eleven body circumferences and six bone diameters as indicated in Figures 3–2 and 3–3, height, and weight were determined for each subject yearly. Circumferences were measured with cloth tape calibrated frequently against a wooden meter stick. A cloth tape was used to avoid compression of underlying skin. Diameters were measured with a broad-blade (¾ inch) anthropometer for comfort and accuracy. Weight was determined with a standard clinical beam balance. Height was measured against a paper wall scale (Iowa Child Welfare Research Station, 1925) with a plastic head level developed for the purpose. Per cent of body fat was calculated as the difference between body weight as measured and lean body weight as calculated from height and diameters.[*]

Rationale for these calculations and more explicit details regarding measurements are discussed by Behnke in the references already cited (1961, 1963a, 1963b) and in a recent companion volume to this report (1972).

Table 3-1 shows the number and range of percent of body fat for each group. These divisions, as already described in Chapter 2, were arbitrarily established. For each sex the 10 percent with the least amount of fat we called "lean," the next fifteen percent "somewhat lean," the middle fifty percent "average," the next fifteen percent "somewhat obese" and the ten percent with the largest amount of fat we called "obese."

We must point out that in our terms "lean body weight" is the weight of the lean body mass and includes an undetermined but probably constant percentage of essential lipids in bone marrow, the central nervous system and other organs. It therefore differs from fat-free weight since it includes the weight of the essential fat.

As in previous work (Behnke, 1961, 1963a, 1963b, 1972),

---

[*] Calculated lean body weight and percent of fat:

$$\text{Females: Lean Body Weight} = \left(\frac{\text{Sum of Diameters}}{83.5}\right)^2 \times \text{Height}^{1.0}$$

$$\text{Males: Lean Body Weight} = \left(\frac{\text{Sum of Diameters}}{54.6}\right)^2 \times \text{Height}^{0.7}$$

$$\text{PerCent Fat} = \frac{W - LBW}{W} \times 100$$

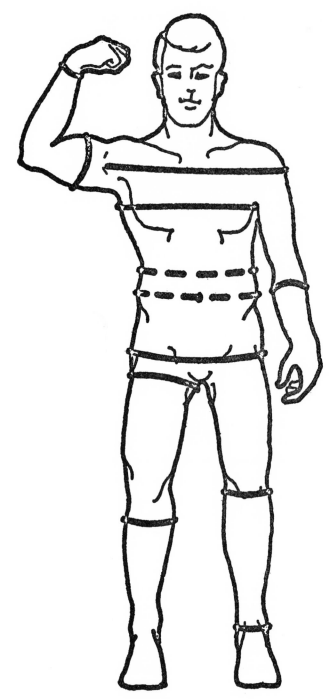

Figure 3–2. Location of Circumference Measurements.

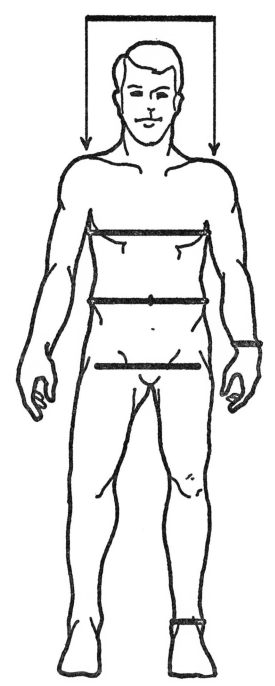

Figure 3–3. Location of Bone Diameter Measurements.

TABLE 3–I
PERCENT BODY FAT CLASSES *

Class Description	MALES Class Range	N	FEMALES Class Range	N
	Ninth Grade			
Lean	Less than +3.25	46	Less than +7.38	52
Somewhat lean	+3.26 to +6.33	69	+7.39 to +11.68	78
Average	+6.34 to +15.14	228	+11.69 to +22.30	259
Somewhat obese	+15.15 to +20.08	69	+22.31 to +26.30	78
Obese	+20.09 plus	46	+26.31 plus	52
		458		519
	Tenth Grade			
Lean	Less than +3.51	45	Less than +6.35	45
Somewhat lean	+3.52 to +6.89	68	+6.36 to +11.56	68
Average	+6.90 to +16.27	228	+11.57 to +21.15	226
Somewhat obese	+16.28 to +21.82	68	+21.16 to +25.90	68
Obese	+21.83 plus	45	+25.91 plus	45
		454		452
	Eleventh Grade			
Lean	Less than +4.51	47	Less than +9.22	42
Somewhat lean	+4.52 to +7.80	70	+9.23 to +14.01	64
Average	+7.81 to +16.60	232	+14.02 to +22.82	212
Somewhat obese	+16.61 to +21.29	70	+22.83 to +27.91	64
Obese	+21.30 plus	47	+27.92 plus	42
		466		424
	Twelfth Grade			
Lean	Less than +4.38	40	Less than +7.30	40
Somewhat lean	+4.39 to +7.65	60	+7.31 to +11.63	61
Average	+7.66 to +16.70	203	+11.64 to +21.49	202
Somewhat obese	+16.71 to +21.94	60	+21.50 to +26.48	61
Obese	+21.95 plus	40	+26.49 plus	40
		403		404

* Fat class ranges based on total students measured each year.

good correlation was achieved between circumferences and weights in all races. The correlation coefficients of the sum of the circumferences divided by a constant ($\epsilon \frac{c}{k}$) to the square root of the weight in kilograms divided by the height in decimeters ($\sqrt{\frac{W}{H}}$) are as follows: (Since our results for each year were similar we are reporting only those of the first year.)

CORRELATION COEFFICIENTS

	Boys	Girls
Caucasian	0.99196	0.98085
Negro	0.99316	0.97818
Oriental	0.99392	0.98209
Unknown	0.99594	0.93973
Total Sample	0.99252	0.98049

Somatograms

In distributing the somatograms to the subjects, the term "body measurement profile" was used. Figure 3–1 is a form similar to the one given to the students. The somatograms shown in Figure 3–1 are those of one boy who became fat between the ages of fourteen and seventeen. This boy was "average" in the ninth grade and obese in the twelfth grade. Note that in the ninth grade his ankles, knees, and wrists were larger than his average and that his biceps, forearms, and chest were considerably smaller. This was rather typical of the teenage boys measured. Since their measurements were compared to adult standards (Behnke, 1961, 1963a, 1963b, 1972), it appears that their skeletal development is somewhat in advance of soft tissue development. After the boy became obese note that his larger measurements are abdomen and thigh, areas in which excess fat is usually deposited.

Differences between means were tested for statistical significance using the standard error of the differences between two means, for large and small size samples, when appropriate.

Size of Error

To estimate the amount of possible error in our procedure, we did a small substudy with two female subjects and one experienced technician. Each of the subjects was measured twenty times over a four-week period (approximately once a day). The technician was not allowed to see any of the previous data. We made no effort to control the time of day of measuring, voiding of urine, or pre- or post-prandial condition of the subjects, since these conditions were not controlled in the main study. The mean and variance of lean body weight and percent of body fat were determined by a straightforward application of the propagation of error formula. Table 3-II shows that the most reproducible of the diameters and accessory measurements are stature, bi-iliac diameter, ankle diameter, weight and bitrochanteric diameter. The most reproducible of the circumferential measurements are the ankle, calf, wrist, and forearm. The least reproducible value is the percent of body fat, as it is calculated from several measurements. Agreement, however, is still acceptable.

TABLE 3-II

MEAN, RANGE AND COEFFICIENT OF VARIATION * OF BODY MEASUREMENTS OF TWO ADULT FEMALES LISTED IN RANK ORDER BY COEFFICIENT OF VARIATION

Diameters (cm), Stature (dm), Weight (kg), Lean Body Weight (kg), and Body Fat (%)

	Subject A				Subject B			
	Label	X	100% Range	CV (%)	Label	X	100% Range	CV (%)
1.	Stature	17.18	17.14– 17.22	0.16	Stature	16.17	16.10–16.25	0.27
2.	Bi-iliac	29.03	28.5 – 29.3	0.61	Bi-iliac	26.88	26.7 –27.2	0.55
3.	Weight	67.18	66.2 – 68.4	0.78	Bitrochanteric	33.30	32.8 –33.7	0.66
4.	Ankle, R	6.16	6.1 – 6.2	0.81	Weight	56.85	56.2 –57.7	0.74
5.	Ankle, L	6.18	6.1 – 6.3	0.89	Ankle, R	6.60	6.5 – 6.7	0.77
6.	Bitrochanteric	34.94	34.1 – 35.3	1.00	Wrist, L	5.08	5.0 – 5.1	0.81
7.	Lean body weight	54.39		1.23	Ankle, L	6.62	6.5 – 6.7	0.83
8.	Biacromial	36.90	36.2 – 37.6	1.34	Lean body weight	48.81		0.98
9.	Wrist, R	4.86	4.8 – 5.0	1.54	Wrist, R	5.18	5.1 – 5.3	1.00
10.	Wrist, L	5.08	4.9 – 5.2	1.67	Chest	25.16	24.4 –25.9	1.50
11.	Chest	25.42	24.2 – 26.4	2.40	Biacromial	36.24	34.5 –37.0	1.58
12.	% body fat	19.03		4.46	% body fat	14.14		7.10

Circumferences (cm)

	Subject A				Subject B			
	Label	X	100% Range	CV (%)	Label	X	100% Range	CV (%)
1.	Ankle, R	20.55	20.4 – 20.8	0.54	Biceps, L	26.63	26.4 –26.8	0.45
2.	Calf, L	35.29	34.9 – 35.8	0.55	Wrist, R	14.96	14.8 –15.1	0.50
2.5					Wrist, R			
2.5					Wrist, L	14.64	14.5 –14.8	0.50
3.	Ankle, L	20.58	20.4 – 20.9	0.59				
4.	Thigh, R	63.62	62.9 – 64.3	0.60				
4.5					Biceps, R	27.47	27.1 –27.7	0.54
4.5					Thigh, L	56.16	55.5 –56.7	0.54
5.5	Forearm, L	23.72	23.4 – 24.0	0.62				
5.5	Forearm, R	23.75	23.4 – 24.0	0.62				
6.					Calf, L	34.50	34.2 –34.9	0.55
7.	Wrist, R	14.93	14.8 – 15.1	0.64	Ankle, R	21.70	21.5 –21.8	0.57
8.	Wrist, L	15.09	14.9 – 15.3	0.69	Shoulder	98.24	97.1 –99.2	0.60
9.	Calf, R	35.82	35.4 – 36.4	0.73	Ankle, L	21.50	21.2 –21.8	0.62
10.	Thigh, L	62.50	61.6 – 63.5	0.79	Buttocks	98.48	97.2 –99.6	0.65
11.	Biceps, R	28.17	27.7 – 28.7	0.83	Forearm, R	24.04	23.8 –24.4	0.67
12.	Lower abdomen	88.42	86.2 – 90.5	0.90	Forearm, L	23.47	23.2 –23.7	0.71
13.	Buttocks	107.01	104.4 –108.8	0.94	Calf, R	34.16	33.7 –34.7	0.78
14.	Shoulder	102.88	101.5 –104.2	1.19	Thigh, R	56.94	56.0 –57.7	0.86
15.	Biceps, L	28.24	27.6 – 28.9	1.26	Knee, R	36.54	35.8 –37.4	0.95
16.	Chest	88.08	86.8 – 91.1	1.31	Knee, L	35.36	34.8 –36.1	1.04
17.	Knee, R	38.62	37.9 – 39.2	1.91	Chest	83.12	81.6 –85.6	1.13
18.	Knee, L	38.04	37.3 – 38.7	1.99	Upper abdomen	66.20	63.9 –68.0	1.57
19.	Upper abdomen	79.18	76.5 – 82.2	2.32	Lower abdomen	78.72	76.4 –80.4	1.66

* Coefficient of Variation is the ratio of the standard deviation to the arithmetic mean expressed in percent; CV = $\dfrac{\sigma}{\bar{x}} \cdot 100.0$

TABLE 3-III

CORRELATION COEFFICIENTS AND MEAN VALUES OF VARIOUS METHODS OF DETERMINING RELATIVE FATNESS

Groups	Age Mean	SD		N	"r"	Anthropometry % Fat X	σ	Observational Rating* On Six Point Scale X	σ
9th Grade Boys	14.49	0.489	Caucasian	188	0.74	11.2	8.00	2.7	1.03
			Negro	75	0.78	11.5	7.93	2.3	1.03
			Oriental	21	0.81	9.1	6.71	2.3	1.02
9th Grade Girls	14.51	0.433	Caucasian	28	0.83	19.6	7.78	3.8	1.07
			Negro	90	0.74	18.0	7.68	3.5	1.00
			Oriental	13	0.42	10.1	6.77	2.7	0.91
12th Grade Boys	17.29	0.450	All	403	0.77	12.6	7.34	2.9	1.08
12th Grade Girls	17.23	0.390	All	404	0.74	16.8	7.94	3.1	0.87

Groups	Age Mean	SD		N	"r"	Anthropometry % Fat X	σ	Wetzel Grid** Rating X	σ
10th Grade Boys	15.32	0.489	All	454	0.81	12.1	7.57	4.9	1.92
10th Grade Girls	15.24	0.432	All	452	0.83	16.4	7.74	5.9	2.07

Groups	Age Mean	SD		N	"r"	Anthropometry % Fat X	σ	Skinfolds (mm) X	σ
10th Grade Girls Skinfolds:	15.24	0.432	Scapular	63	0.61	16.7	7.44	14.01	6.20
			Triceps	63	0.59			18.39	5.74
			Sum of 2	63	0.64			32.41	11.16

TABLE 3-III (Cont'd.)

		GROUPS				METHODS			
		Mean Age	SD	N	"r"	Wetzel Grid² Rating X	σ	Skinfolds (mm) X	σ
10th Grade Girls		15.24	0.432						
Skinfolds:	Scapular			63	0.70			14.01	6.20
	Triceps			63	0.79	5.9	1.90	18.39	5.74
	Sum of 2			63	0.80			32.41	11.16
						Anthropometry % Fat X	σ	Skinfolds (mm) X	σ
11th Grade Girls		16.23	0.378						
Skinfolds:	Scapular			83	0.729			14.78	6.70
	Triceps			83	0.768			19.98	6.71
	Thorax			83	0.674	15.4	9.42	17.37	7.72
	Abdomen			83	0.697			26.19	10.41
	Sum of 4			83	0.785			78.32	28.66

* Rating on a simple six point scale with 3 indicating a normal amount of fatness, values above 3 denoting increased corpulence, and values below 3 indicating varying degrees of leanness.
** Wetzel Grid rating scale: 1 = (B₄) poor, 2 = (B₃) borderline, 3 = (B₂) fair, 4-5-6 = (B₁, M, A₁) good, 7-8 = (A₂, A₃) stocky, 9 = (A₄) obese.

TABLE 3–IV

CORRELATION COEFFICIENTS AND MEAN VALUES OF DETERMINING
LEAN BODY WEIGHT BY SEVERAL METHODS

Groups *		N	"r"	Methods			
				Anthropometry Lean Body Weight (kg)		*K40* Lean Body Weight (kg)	
				X̄	σ	X̄	σ
Boys	All	89	0.77	55.2	6.49	55.7	7.94
	Caucasian	54	0.74	55.7	6.29	54.7	7.19
	Negro	24	0.85	55.9	5.94	59.7	8.06
	Oriental	11	0.91	50.7	6.89	51.9	7.85
Girls	All	93	0.65	47.3	5.16	40.9	5.83
	Caucasian	59	0.64	47.9	5.02	41.3	5.77
	Negro	25	0.69	47.1	5.51	42.2	4.98
	Oriental	9	0.46	43.4	2.82	35.0	4.88
				Anthropometry Lean Body Weight (kg)		*Specific Gravity* Lean Body Weight (kg)	
				X̄	σ	X̄	σ
Boys	All	89	0.84	55.2	6.49	55.9	8.60
	Caucasian	54	0.85	55.7	6.29	55.5	8.28
	Negro	24	0.83	55.9	5.94	59.1	8.91
	Oriental	11	0.90	50.7	6.89	50.9	6.29
Girls	All	93	0.74	47.3	5.16	41.1	5.56
	Caucasian	59	0.72	47.9	5.02	41.2	5.22
	Negro	25	0.83	47.1	5.51	42.2	6.25
	Oriental	9	−0.005	43.4	2.82	37.0	3.40
				Specific Gravity Lean Body Weight (kg)		*K40* Lean Body Weight (kg)	
				X̄	σ	X̄	σ
Boys	All	89	0.88	55.9	8.60	55.7	7.94
	Caucasian	54	0.86	55.5	8.28	54.7	7.19
	Negro	24	0.89	59.1	8.91	59.7	8.06
	Oriental	11	0.90	50.9	6.29	51.9	7.85
Girls	All	93	0.72	41.1	5.56	40.9	5.83
	Caucasian	59	0.72	41.2	5.22	41.3	5.77
	Negro	25	0.69	42.2	6.25	42.2	4.98
	Oriental	9	0.55	37.0	3.40	35.0	4.88

* Subjects were approximately 16 years of age.

The least reproducible circumferences are chest, knee, and upper
and lower abdomen.

Comparison with Other Methods

Tables 3-III and 3-IV show the correlations between our
method of assessing percent of body fat and various other methods of determining relative obesity with various subsamples.
(See Behnke and Wilmore, 1972, for details of methods other
than skinfolds.) Each series of skinfolds was done by the same
technician using a Lange constant pressure caliper.

The correlations between lean body weight as determined by
anthropometry and as determined by radioactive potassium and
specific gravity are higher for boys than girls. Apparently girls,
no matter how lean they appear, are not as dense and lean as
boys. The leanest girl had a body weight very closely in agree-

ment with lean body weight as determined anthropometrically but not as determined by other methods. Therefore, the term "minimal weight" would be more appropriate than lean body weight (as determined anthropometrically) when referring to females. This finding that girls even at minimal weight have more fat tissue than boys may have broad clinical applications. The Negro boys had a higher lean body weight as measured by radioactive potassium counting and specific gravity than lean body weight as measured by the anthropometric method. This indicates a heavier skeletal structure or more or denser muscle mass.

Body Measurements

Table A-I in Appendix A indicates the quintile ranges for all four years, including all measurements taken. It suggests that normal ranges for body fat by the method we used might be considered to be from about 10 to 15 percent for boys and from 15 to 20 percent for girls. The distribution of percentage of body fat for each of the four grades is shown in Figure 3–2.

Table A-II in Appendix A shows the mean values obtained for the various body measurements of all subjects for each grade. While standard deviations in the case of some measurements were sufficiently large to make differences between races statistically insignificant, it is nevertheless interesting to observe that there is a consistent trend for measurements of Caucasian boys to exceed those of Negroes and for those of Negroes to be greater than those of Orientals in the 9th grade. The exception is the bi-iliac measurement which was larger for Oriental boys than Negro boys. By the following year, Negro boys tended to exceed Caucasians in biceps, forearm, and chest measurements and in percent of body fat. These differences held for the third and fourth year as well. Again, Oriental boys had a larger bi-iliac measurement than the Negroes, but were smaller in other measurements than the Negroes and Caucasians.

In the case of girls, on the other hand, Negroes already tended to exceed Caucasians in all but hip, lower extremity and stature measurements in the ninth grade. They continued to have smaller hip diameters but larger abdominal circumferences, greater weight and higher percent of body fat throughout the remainder of the study. Oriental girls had smaller measurements than the other two groups throughout the four years of the study. Differences of statistical significance are indicated in Table A-II, Appendix A.

Tanner (1964) has shown significant differences in body conformation and composition between athletes of different races.

The percent of body fat, while not significantly different consistently at the 0.01 level of all four grades, did show some significant differences at both the 0.05 and 0.01 levels. For the boys the differences were significant at either level for four grades for the Oriental to the Negro boys, and for Caucasian to Negro for the last three grades. The Negro boys had a higher percent of body fat than the other boys. However, this finding might be misleading due to the higher lean body weight of Negro boys when measured by body density or radioactive potassium counting than when measured by anthropometry. The higher percent of body fat of the Negro girls was significantly different from that of the Caucasian girls for four grades at the 0.01 level. The Negro girls also had a higher percent of fat than the Oriental girls, significant at the 0.01 level for three grades and at the 0.05 level for one grade. The Caucasian girls had a significantly (0.05 level) higher percent of body fat than the Oriental girls in the ninth and eleventh grades.

The Oriental girls differed from the Negro and Caucasian girls in more of their measurements for the first three grades of the study than they did in the twelfth grade, suggesting a possible difference in age of maturation. When we asked our subjects the age at which they experienced their first menses, we discovered that the Caucasian girls reported a mean of 12.7 years, the Negro girls a mean of 12.3 years, and the Oriental girls a mean of 12.7 years. These means indicate only that the Negro girls matured a bit earlier than the other two groups. The difference between the Caucasian and Negro girls is statistically significant.

Prevalence of Obesity

A method of assessing obesity is to select arbitrary cut-off points in amount of body fat and to compare the numbers that fall into these ranges from year to year. To classify our obese

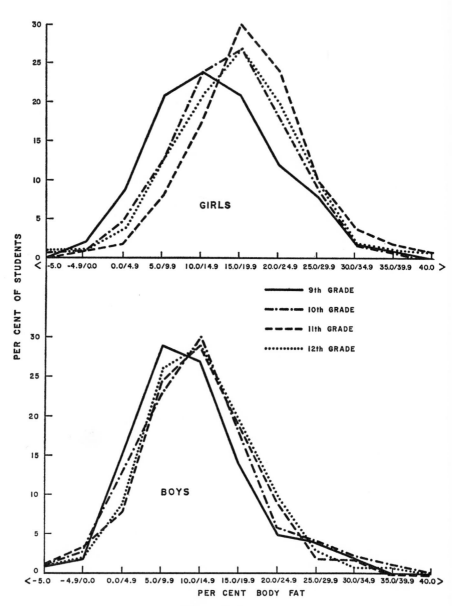

Figure 3–4.

subjects, we selected the cut-off point of over 20 percent body fat for boys and 25 percent for girls. While these cut-off points were arbitrary, they do relate to the previously mentioned normal ranges indicated in Table A-I in Appendix A. Using these ranges, we found little difference in the percent of boys who fell into the obese classifications from year to year. For the girls, there was an increase up to the third year, and a drop in the fourth year. (See Table 3-V.)

Growth

Table 3-VI shows the values obtained each year for the subjects who were measured all four years. The mean values of all body measurements of this longitudinal sample were not significantly different (0.05 level) from the means of the total sample measured each year.

Although boys showed more significant changes from grade to grade than girls, the pattern shows that both sexes were growing, the boys more rapidly.

The boys' consistent increase in diameters, lean body weight, and stature indicates rapid skeletal growth which seemed to slow down during the eleventh to the twelfth grade when their per cent of body fat increased significantly. The increasing circumferences of their forearms, calves, and biceps indicates that the boys' musculature as well as skeletal size was increasing.

The girls increased in lean body weight, stature and some diameters from ninth to twelfth grade, although all increases were smaller than those of the boys. Female calf, biceps and forearm circumferences increased slightly from ninth to twelfth grade, which may indicate a growth in musculature during these years. This small, but continuing, growth of the girls may mean that girls' as well as boys' nutritional needs continue to increase throughout the high school years. Their percent of body fat increased (0.01 level of significance) from the tenth grade to the eleventh grade, decreasing (0.05 level of significance) from the eleventh grade to the twelfth grade. This made us wonder if perhaps the first change was a normal development and the subsequent decrease a result of voluntary caloric restriction by many of the subjects.

Using the radioactive potassium counting method, Forbes

TABLE 3–V

PREVALENCE OF OBESITY

	Ninth Grade %	N	Tenth Grade %	N	Eleventh Grade %	N	Twelfth Grade %	N
Boys								
Mild obesity (20% body fat)	5	23	6	25	9	44	9	37
Marked obesity (25% body fat)	6	27	7	29	5	22	5	20
Girls								
Mild obesity (25% body fat)	8	41	9	42	10	42	10	41
Marked obesity (30% body fat)	3	16	3	17	7	27	4	16

TABLE 3–VIA

CIRCUMFERENCES, DIAMETERS, AND ACCESSORY INFORMATION, LONGITUDINAL SAMPLE

	Ninth Grade $\bar{X}$	σ	Boys (N = 227) Tenth Grade $\bar{X}$	σ	Eleventh Grade $\bar{X}$	σ	Twelfth Grade $\bar{X}$	σ
Circumferences (cm)								
Abdomen	69.54 †	7.818	70.53	7.899	72.24	7.641	73.98 †	7.984
Ankle	21.44 †	1.678	21.83	1.594	22.15	1.480	22.04 †	1.459
Biceps	26.97 †	3.165	28.20	3.093	29.51 *	2.757	30.54 *†	2.855
Buttocks	84.18 *†	7.839	86.46 *	7.376	88.51 *	6.649	90.02 †	6.900
Calf	33.37 †	2.982	33.99 *	2.799	34.89 *	2.686	35.22 †	2.676
Chest	81.64 *†	7.666	84.29 *	7.365	87.39	6.419	88.83 †	6.703
Forearm	23.89 *†	2.035	24.75 *	1.904	25.56 *	1.699	26.22 *†	1.704
Knee	34.46 †	2.696	34.99	2.510	35.45	2.281	35.44 †	2.238
Shoulder	98.73 *†	8.028	103.00 *	7.619	106.60 *	6.594	108.94 *†	6.407
Thigh	50.08 *†	6.066	51.70 *	5.881	52.73	5.596	53.44 †	5.407
Wrist	15.74 *†	0.943	16.04 *	0.851	16.32 *	0.781	16.49 †	0.813
Diameters (cm)								
Ankle	13.78 *†	0.738	14.10 *	0.722	14.13	0.720	14.24 †	0.757
Biacromial	36.43 *†	2.438	37.57 *	2.250	38.68 *	1.949	39.73 *†	1.794
Bi-iliac	25.58 *†	1.981	26.34 *	1.911	26.99 *	1.809	27.34 †	1.887
Bitrochanteric	29.63 *†	2.298	30.58 *	2.075	31.43 *	1.753	31.95 *†	1.740
Chest	25.66 *†	1.999	26.55 *	1.956	27.13 *	1.740	27.79 *†	1.736
Wrist	10.67 *†	0.700	10.95 *	0.627	11.19 *	0.603	11.28 *†	0.627
Accessory Information								
Stature (dm)	16.58 *†	0.835	16.99 *	0.766	17.36 *	0.713	17.57 *†	0.717
Lean body wt. (kg)	48.46 *†	7.395	52.25 *	6.894	55.52 *	6.201	58.06 *†	6.194
Weight (kg)	55.52 *†	12.215	59.83 *	11.938	64.06 *	11.342	67.13 *†	11.691
% body fat	11.54 †	7.603	11.52	7.672	12.30 *	7.931	12.47 *†	7.918
Age (years)	14.49	0.489	15.32	0.489	16.36	0.508	17.29	0.450

NOTE: Abdomen circumference represents the mean of upper and lower portions of the abdomen. Ankle, biceps, calf, forearm, knee, thigh and wrist circumferences represent the mean of the right and left sides. Ankle and wrist diameters represent the sum of the right and left sides.
* Significant differences (0.01 level), from grade to grade.
† Significant differences (0.01 level) from grades 9 to 12.

TABLE 3–VIB

CIRCUMFERENCES, DIAMETERS, AND ACCESSORY INFORMATION,
LONGITUDINAL SAMPLE

	GIRLS (N = 254)							
	NINTH GRADE		TENTH GRADE		ELEVENTH GRADE		TWELFTH GRADE	
	X̄	σ	X̄	σ	X̄	σ	X̄	σ
Circumferences (cm)								
Abdomen	71.02 †	5.874	72.18	6.246	69.59	6.267	72.62 †	6.473
Ankle	21.15	1.379	21.05	1.416	21.27	1.371	21.38	1.411
Biceps	25.89 †	2.316	25.85 *	2.436	26.68 *	2.519	26.87 †	2.644
Buttocks	91.75 †	6.127	92.89	6.237	93.26	6.188	94.39 †	6.273
Calf	34.10 †	2.512	34.15 *	2.601	34.77 *	2.495	35.04 †	2.593
Chest	82.15 *†	5.163	83.47 *‡	5.209	83.34 *‡	5.141	84.69 *†	5.334
Forearm	22.87	1.482	22.56 *	1.669	22.95 *	1.560	23.57 *†	1.588
Knee	34.77 *†	2.197	35.91 *	2.425	35.98	2.362	36.35 †	2.498
Shoulder	96.15 *†	5.520	98.15 *	5.884	98.04	5.991	98.96 †	5.696
Thigh	55.85	5.210	56.53	4.979	57.19	4.706	56.22	5.056
Wrist	15.11	0.693	14.97	0.780	15.20	0.723	15.19	0.750
Diameters (cm)								
Ankle	12.19 †	0.617	12.26	0.551	12.15 *	0.573	12.55 *†	0.581
Biacromial	35.31 *†	1.784	35.75 *	1.857	35.74	1.753	35.85 †	1.815
Bi-iliac	26.14 *†	1.622	26.78 *‡	1.768	26.93 *‡	1.679	27.74 *†	1.839
Bitrochanteric	30.63 †	1.773	30.81	1.806	30.97 *	1.641	31.46 *†	1.754
Chest	25.13	1.573	25.25	1.535	24.45	1.438	24.59	1.495
Wrist	9.74	0.525	9.90	0.543	9.60	0.523	10.03	0.539
Accessory Information								
Stature (dm)	16.16 †	0.643	16.25	0.635	16.34	0.640	16.39 †	0.642
Lean body wt. (kg)	45.04 *†	5.264	46.35 *‡	5.359	46.00 *‡	5.085	47.74 *†	5.496
Weight (kg)	54.27 †	8.203	55.43	8.654	56.67	8.764	57.75 †	9.155
% body fat	16.34	7.096	15.62 *	7.649	18.04	7.810	16.54	7.931
Age (years)	14.51	0.433	15.24	0.432	16.23	0.378	17.23	0.390

NOTE: Abdomen circumference represents the mean of upper and lower portions of the abdomen. Ankle, biceps, calf, forearm, knee, thigh and wrist circumferences represent the mean of the right and left sides. Ankle and wrist diameters represent the sum of the right and left sides.
* Significant differences (0.01 level) from grade to grade.
† Significant differences (0.01 level) from grades 9 to 12.
‡ Insignificant differences between grades 10 and 11.

(1964) found that lean body mass reaches a maximum in males at eighteen to twenty years of age and in females at fifteen to sixteen years of age. Similarly, there was a large increase in lean body weight of our boys up to age seventeen. However, we also found small increases in lean body weight for the girls in our study up to age seventeen.

Skeletal Differences

Since there were significant differences in many of the body measurements, including stature, between the various racial groups, we thought these differences might be affected by differences in stature. To give a clearer indication of body conformation, by shape rather than size, we divided diameter measurements in centimeters by stature measurements in decimeters. Table 3-IX shows racial differences in these ratios. Negro boys and girls have smaller bi-iliac and bitrochanteric to stature ratios than Oriental or Caucasian boys and girls. Caucasian boys and girls have smaller biacromial to stature ratios than do Oriental or Negro boys and girls. Oriental boys and girls tend to have larger diameter to stature ratios than do the other boys and girls.

Body Fat Groups. We also applied these ratios to our arbitrary classification of degree of fatness. Table 3-X shows the stature, and diameter to stature, ratios of boys and girls in these different fat classifications. Data for ninth and twelfth grade only are shown since data for all four grades were similar.

More significant differences between fat classes appear for the girls than for the boys. The obese boys tend to be the tallest, particularly in the ninth grade, the differences in height becoming progressively less the next three grades. This pattern fits the classical picture of the fast growing, early maturing boys being inclined to obesity. The ninth grade was the only one in which any significant differences appeared in the stature of the boys. In that year the only significant difference was obese boys to average boys. The girls, on the other hand, present a different picture. In all grades the lean and somewhat lean girls were taller than the other girls. Did this height indicate that the lean girls matured early?

Menstrual Age. We compared ages of the beginning of menstruation for the various twelfth grade fat classes. We found that the mean age was 12.9 years for the lean girls, 12.7 years for the somewhat lean, 12.5 years for the average, 12.6 years for the somewhat obese and 12.2 years for the obese girls. This indicated that the lean and somewhat lean girls were later in maturing than were the obese girls, and that the average and somewhat obese girls were in between. The difference between the lean and obese girls was statistically significant at the 0.05 level. This later maturation for the lean girls is especially striking since they tended to be taller than others throughout their high school years.

Body Fat Groups Divided by Race. The mean values for some of the diameter to stature ratios for the Negro and Oriental boys and girls differed from the overall average fat classes for all four grades (Table 3-VII and 3-VIII). To make more detailed comparisons, therefore, we further subdivided our subjects into fat classes by racial groups. Table 3-IX shows the results, presenting data for the ninth grade only. The wrist and ankle to

TABLE 3-VII

RATIOS OF SOME BODY DIAMETERS TO STATURE CLASSIFIED BY SEX, SCHOOL YEAR, AND RACE

School Year / Race	N	Biacromial/Stature X̄	σ	Bi-iliac/Stature X̄	σ	Bitrochanteric/Stature X̄	σ
Boys							
Ninth grade							
Caucasian	267	2.18 *	0.106	1.56	0.080	1.80	0.084
Negro	137	2.21	0.117	1.49 *	0.085	1.75 *	0.097
Oriental	43	2.25	0.110	1.58	0.083	1.80	0.090
Tenth grade							
Caucasian	258	2.19 *	0.117	1.57	0.073	1.81	0.077
Negro	152	2.23	0.102	1.50 *	0.082	1.77 *	0.090
Oriental	36	2.26	0.108	1.58	0.081	1.82	0.085
Eleventh grade							
Caucasian	250	2.20 *	0.115	1.58	0.078	1.82	0.076
Negro	168	2.25	0.099	1.50 *	0.073	1.77 *	0.076
Oriental	37	2.29	0.109	1.59	0.088	1.83	0.065
Twelfth grade							
Caucasian	224	2.23 *	0.107	1.58	0.082	1.83	0.077
Negro	140	2.29	0.097	1.50 *	0.077	1.78 *	0.081
Oriental	35	2.33	0.105	1.60	0.086	1.84	0.067
Girls							
Ninth grade							
Caucasian	316	2.16 *	0.118	1.63	0.110	1.90	0.115
Negro	147	2.21	0.098	1.59 *	0.110	1.89	0.122
Oriental	42	2.21	0.088	1.65	0.105	1.91	0.102
Tenth grade							
Caucasian	268	2.18 *	0.100	1.67	0.102	1.91	0.100
Negro	142	2.22	0.107	1.60 *	0.114	1.88 *	0.102
Oriental	34	2.24	0.099	1.68	0.076	1.91	0.084
Eleventh grade							
Caucasian	246	2.17 *	0.091	1.67	0.086	1.90	0.085
Negro	139	2.22	0.102	1.58 *	0.100	1.88 *	0.107
Oriental	36	2.21	0.094	1.70	0.093	1.92	0.090
Twelfth grade							
Caucasian	245	2.17 *	0.095	1.71	0.095	1.92	0.095
Negro	117	2.21	0.110	1.64 *	0.110	1.91	0.110
Oriental	37	2.23	0.084	1.74	0.121	1.95	0.106

* Significant difference (0.05 level) from other two means within grade, sex.

TABLE 3-VIII

MEAN VALUES OF STATURE, AND DIAMETER TO STATURE RATIOS OF HIGH SCHOOL STUDENTS CLASSIFIED BY SEX, GRADE, AND BODY FAT GROUP

	N	Stature (dm)	Bitrochanteric/Stature	Wrist/Stature	Ankle/Stature	Bi-iliac/Stature	Biacromial/Stature
Boys							
Ninth Grade							
Lean	45	16.66	1.76	0.64	0.82	1.55	2.20
Somewhat lean	68	16.59	1.76	0.64	0.83	1.54	2.19
Average	228	16.53	1.76	0.64	0.83	1.52	2.19
Somewhat obese	70	16.73	1.81 †	0.65	0.84	1.54	2.21
Obese	46	16.84	1.89 ‡	0.63	0.84	1.62 ‡	2.24 †
Twelfth Grade							
Lean	40	17.71	1.80	0.64	0.81	1.56	2.26
Somewhat lean	58	17.74	1.79	0.64	0.80	1.53	2.23
Average	205	17.58	1.81	0.64	0.81	1.54	2.26
Somewhat obese	59	17.76	1.82	0.65	0.82	1.54	2.25
Obese	41	17.73	1.91 ‡	0.65	0.83 †	1.63 ‡	2.29
Girls							
Ninth Grade							
Lean	52	16.37 †	1.86	0.60	0.75	1.59	2.15
Somewhat lean	77	16.27 †	1.86	0.60	0.75	1.60	2.15
Average	259	16.17	1.90	0.60	0.76	1.61	2.18
Somewhat obese	78	15.95	1.95 †	0.61	0.77 †	1.65 †	2.20 †
Obese	53	16.10	2.01 ‡	0.62 †	0.77 †	1.72 ‡	2.23 ‡
Twelfth Grade							
Lean	39	16.60 †	1.88	0.61	0.76	1.69	2.18
Somewhat lean	60	16.54 †	1.88	0.60	0.76	1.67	2.16
Average	203	16.37	1.90	0.61	0.76	1.67	2.18
Somewhat obese	61	16.24	1.95 †	0.62	0.78 †	1.70	2.20
Obese	41	16.22	2.03 ‡	0.62 †	0.79 †	1.78 ‡	2.26 †

† Significantly larger (0.05 level) than some other body fat groups.
‡ Significantly larger (0.05 level) than all other body fat groups.

TABLE 3-IX

MEAN VALUES OF STATURE AND DIAMETER TO STATURE RATIOS OF NINTH-GRADE STUDENTS CLASSIFIED BY SEX, RACE, AND BODY FAT GROUP

	Boys					Girls				
	Boys N	Stature (dm)	Bitrochanteric/Stature	Bi-iliac/Stature	Biacromial/Stature	Girls N	Stature (dm)	Bitrochanteric/Stature	Bi-iliac/Stature	Biacromial/Stature
Caucasian										
Lean	29	16.98	1.79	1.57	2.19	34	16.58 †	1.87	1.60	2.14
Somewhat lean	41	16.86	1.76	1.55	2.17	47	16.34	1.87	1.60	2.12
Average	127	16.73	1.78	1.54	2.18	163	16.26	1.90	1.62	2.17
Somewhat obese	43	16.89	1.82	1.56	2.19	42	16.09	1.96	1.68	2.17
Obese	27	17.14	1.89 ‡	1.64 ‡	2.21	30	16.05	2.00 ‡	1.73 †	2.22 ‡
Negro										
Lean	11	16.17	1.69	1.46	2.18	7	16.21	1.81	1.55	2.17
Somewhat lean	16	16.50	1.74	1.51	2.22	18	16.57 †	1.81	1.54	2.17
Average	73	16.40	1.73	1.48	2.20	77	16.13	1.87	1.57	2.21
Somewhat obese	24	16.54	1.78	1.49	2.23	24	16.01	1.94 †‡	1.62	2.22
Obese	13	16.32	1.88 ‡	1.58 †	2.25	21	16.16	2.02 ‡	1.72 ‡	2.24
Oriental										
Lean	5	15.90	1.79	1.61	2.29	9	15.75	1.83	1.59	2.16
Somewhat lean	11	15.72	1.80	1.57	2.24	10	15.55	1.90	1.64	2.20
Average	23	15.92	1.79	1.56	2.23	13	15.56	1.95	1.70	2.25
Somewhat obese	0			—		9	15.36	1.96	1.64	2.23
Obese	4	16.96	1.92	1.65	2.38	1	15.92	1.97	1.76	2.35

† Significantly larger (0.05 level) than some other body fat groups within sex and race.
‡ Significantly larger (0.05 level) than all other body fat groups within sex and race.

stature ratios are not included since there were few differences. Since the sample sizes for the Orientals, both boys and girls, were so small, statistical analysis was not done on those groups.

The most consistent significant differences occur between obese or somewhat obese and other groups in the bitrochanteric to stature ratio, closely followed by the bi-iliac to stature ratio. The biacromial to stature ratio differences are consistently significant for Caucasian girls only.

In comparing our findings to those of Seltzer and Mayer (1964), we seem to confirm their observations on obese and nonobese Caucasian girls. Obese girls have broader bones for unit of body height than do the nonobese. We found this true also for obese and nonobese boys, although the trend is not as well defined. However, the opposite is not true for the lean and somewhat lean subjects in our study since they do not have significantly smaller diameter to stature ratios than do the average subjects.

Predicting Obesity

Can any of these observed differences be used to predict obesity? We selected the subjects who had become obese from the ninth to the twelfth grade. There were only six boys and twelve girls classified as obese in the twelfth grade who were not so classified in the ninth grade. We compared the selected subjects' stature and diameter to stature ratios (Table 3-X) with the same values for the groups in Table 3-IX.

Boy number one was in the tallest 20 percent of the entire sample of boys. His larger than average bi-iliac to stature ratio, biacromial to stature ratio, and bitrochanteric to stature ratio might indeed be predictive of his coming obesity. Of the four Caucasian boys who became obese by the twelfth grade from being somewhat obese in the ninth grade, three were quite tall. Only one was shorter than the mean height of all the groups of Caucasian boys, in fact, in the shortest 20 percent of all the boys. The short boy had quite large diameter to stature ratios; the tallest boy (number five) had smaller diameter to stature ratios than the mean for any group of Caucasian boys with the exception of his biacromial to stature ratio. Perhaps his unusual height had an

TABLE 3-X

NINTH-GRADE STATURE AND DIAMETER TO STATURE RATIOS OF INDIVIDUALS WHO BECAME OBESE BETWEEN NINTH AND TWELFTH GRADES

Subject	Sex	Race	Ninth-Grade Fat Class	Stature (dm)	Bitrochanteric/ Stature	Bi-iliac/ Stature	Biacromial/ Stature
1	Boy	Caucasian	"Average"	17.40 **	1.81 *	1.59 *	2.20 *
2	Boy	Caucasian	"Somewhat Obese"	15.76	2.00 **	1.71 **	2.54 **
3	Boy	Caucasian	"Somewhat Obese"	17.56 **	1.87 *	1.61	2.21 *
4	Boy	Caucasian	"Somewhat Obese"	17.72 **	1.92 **	1.58	2.31 **
5	Boy	Caucasian	"Somewhat Obese"	18.52 **	1.62	1.46	2.20
6	Boy	Negro	"Somewhat Obese"	17.24 **	1.90 **	1.51	2.32 **
7	Girl	Caucasian	"Average"	16.63	1.95 *	1.66	2.20 *
8	Girl	Caucasian	"Somewhat Obese"	15.36	2.00 *	1.76 **	2.13
9	Girl	Caucasian	"Somewhat Obese"	16.55	2.04 **	1.80 **	2.26 **
10	Girl	Caucasian	"Somewhat Obese"	15.15	1.92	1.56	2.19
11	Girl	Caucasian	"Somewhat Obese"	14.78	1.93	1.70	2.44 **
12	Girl	Negro	"Average"	15.98	1.86	1.48	2.00
13	Girl	Negro	"Average"	16.30	2.03 **	1.69 *	2.22
14	Girl	Negro	"Average"	16.84	1.84	1.58	2.26 **
15	Girl	Negro	"Average"	15.86	1.74	1.49	2.18
16	Girl	Negro	"Somewhat Obese"	15.77	1.96	1.62	2.28 **
17	Girl	Negro	"Somewhat Obese"	16.05	2.10 *	1.66	2.32 **
18	Girl	Negro	"Somewhat Obese"	15.84	1.98	1.52	2.20

* Comparable with ninth-grade value for next higher fat class by sex and race.
** Higher than any ninth-grade fat class by sex and race.

unduly large influence on these ratios. Possibly the larger than average height of all but one of these boys was in itself an indication that they were likely to become obese. However, with the exception of the tallest boy, they did show a broader bone structure than the mean value for the group in which they belonged in the ninth grade.

There seemed to be no one clear-cut index to indicate that the somewhat obese Caucasian girls in the ninth grade would become obese by the twelfth grade. However, the one Caucasian girl who was average and became obese did have a large biacromial to stature ratio.

Of the seven Negro girls who became obese, the four who were average in the ninth grade showed no pattern of stature or diameter to stature ratios that might be indicative of their coming obesity. Of the three Negro girls who became obese in the twelfth grade from somewhat obese in the ninth grade, all were shorter than the mean value of stature for all the Negro girls. Other than their height there seemed to be no index that might be predictive.

Our observations on this rather small group of subjects might indicate that taller boys with broad bones are the most inclined to become obese, while girls' broad bone structure is not necessarily a predictive factor in obesity development.

Relationship of Environmental and Genetic Factors to Body Composition

Our data do not solve the controversy of whether obesity is primarily environmental or genetic in origin. We did, however, find associations between obesity and such factors as socioeconomic group, ethnic origin, and fatness of parents.

To determine if there was a relationship between socioeconomic level and percent of body fat, we grouped students each year by mean family income of the census tract which they occupied, using the 1960 United States census figures of family income from Berkeley, California (U.S. Census of Population, 1960) as explained in Chapter 2. Table 3-XI shows percent of body fat by socioeconomic level for all years of the study. The subjects in the lower socioeconomic group tended to have a

TABLE 3-XI

MEAN PER CENT BODY FAT OF NINTH-, TENTH-, ELEVENTH-, AND TWELFTH-GRADE STUDENTS AS CLASSIFIED BY SOCIOECONOMIC LEVEL * (CENSUS TRACT OCCUPIED)

Socioeconomic Level	Ninth Grade						Tenth Grade					
	Boys			Girls			Boys			Girls		
	$\bar{X}$		N	$\bar{X}$		N	$\bar{X}$		N	$\bar{X}$		N
Lower third	12.8 †	6.92	57	19.1 †‡	7.61	48	13.9 †	7.37	60	18.3 ††	9.25	50
Middle third	11.9	7.90	236	16.8 †	7.88	287	12.7	7.96	248	16.9 †	7.67	256
Upper third	9.2 †	6.24	129	15.8 ‡	6.70	159	9.9 †	6.36	124	14.8 ‡	7.13	137

Socioeconomic Level	Eleventh Grade						Twelfth Grade					
	Boys			Girls			Boys			Girls		
	$\bar{X}$		N	$\bar{X}$		N	$\bar{X}$		N	$\bar{X}$		N
Lower third	14.9 †	6.06	64	20.9 †‡	7.67	43	14.2 †	6.85	53	18.4	8.27	49
Middle third	12.9	7.89	256	18.3 †	7.70	243	12.8	7.78	207	17.0	8.01	213
Upper third	10.7 †	6.48	132	17.6 ‡	6.99	130	11.3 †	6.76	123	16.2	7.80	134

† or ‡ Significant differences within each sex, each year between groups so marked (0.05 level).

* *U.S. Census of Population: 1960*, California (Tuddenham and Snyder, 1954)—Table 76 "Income in 1959 of Families and Persons, and Weeks Worked in 1959 for Standard Metropolitan Statistical Areas, Urbanized Areas, and Urban Places of 10,000 and More; 1960," Urban Places—Berkeley.

Lower third: Under $1,000 to $5,110
Middle third: $5,111 to $8,586
Upper third: $8,587 and over

higher percent of body fat than subjects in the upper socioeconomic groups. That this tendency was not as marked for twelfth-grade girls may indicate some deliberate change in habits on the part of those girls in the lower socioeconomic group during their high school years in an effort to become slimmer.

However, the most reliable estimation of socioeconomic class is obtained by a three-factor index (Hollingshead and Redlich, 1958) using education, job and residence. At this date there are no recent cluster analyses of Berkeley census tracts available for this kind of classification. Therefore, we used the two-factor index method of Hollingshead (1957) which uses education and employment rankings to supplement the material obtained by census tract classification. Data on parents' occupation and education were obtained from mailed questionnaires while the students were in the twelfth grade. Table 3-XII shows the results of

TABLE 3–XII

MEAN PER CENT OF BODY FAT OF TWELFTH-GRADE STUDENTS GROUPED INTO HOLLINGSHEAD SOCIAL CLASSES *

Social Class	Boys			Girls		
	$\bar{X}$	σ	N	$\bar{X}$	σ	N
I	10.7	6.13	68	16.0	7.84	74
II	11.4	7.62	30	14.8	7.62	27
III	14.0	6.94	62	14.2	7.82	60
IV	13.9	7.03	54	18.1	7.79	70
V	13.6	10.02	28	18.8	7.16	28

* Hodges and Krehl, 1965.

this analysis. Class I indicates the highest rating; Class V indicates the lowest rating. For the boys Class I has a significantly (0.05 level) lower percent of body fat than classes III, IV, and V. Classes II and III of the girls have a significantly lower percent of body fat than Classes IV and V. While not statistically significant, the Class I girls have a higher percent of body fat than the girls in Classes II and III. The significant differences between socioeconomic groups, determined in two different ways, indicate that those teenagers in the lower socioeconomic groups did have a tendency to be more obese than the more privileged groups.

However, the socioeconomic group may be somewhat dependent on ethnic origin and ethnic origin may involve genetic, socioeconomic, and other environmental factors. Table 3-XIII shows the ethnic distribution in each of the social classes. This table clearly shows that the lower classes were composed of a disproportionate number of Negroes. Orientals, also, tended to fall in the lower socioeconomic groups but not nearly to the extent that the Negroes did. Table 3-XIV shows that the Negro boys

TABLE 3–XIII

PERCENT RACE IN EACH CLASS OF TWELFTH-GRADE STUDENTS GROUPED INTO HOLLINGSHEAD SOCIAL CLASSES *

| | *Total N* | PER CENT OF TOTAL | | | | |
		Caucasian	*Negro*	*Oriental*	*Other*	*Total Per Cent*
Boys						
Class I	68	89.7	2.9	7.4	—	100.0
Class II	30	93.3	6.7	—	—	100.0
Class III	62	72.6	11.3	16.1	—	100.0
Class IV	54	46.3	35.2	13.0	5.5	100.0
Class V	28	35.7	53.6	10.7	—	100.0
Girls						
Class I	74	93.2	—	6.8	—	100.0
Class II	27	85.2	7.4	7.4	—	100.0
Class III	60	76.7	10.0	13.3	—	100.0
Class IV	70	50.0	30.0	18.6	1.4	100.0
Class V	28	17.9	71.4	7.1	3.6	100.0

* Hodges and Krehl, 1965.

and girls had more, and the Oriental boys and girls had less, of a tendency toward obesity than the Caucasians. These tendencies for the Negroes to be fatter, the Orientals to be thinner, for those in the lower socioeconomic classes to be fatter and for both Negroes and Orientals to fall into the lower socioeconomic classes, when combined may indicate that the tendency to obesity is more strongly related to ethnic factors than it is to socioeconomic factors. Ethnicity, while genetically determined, also strongly influences environment.

Other differences that were observed may indicate that genetic factors may be related to obesity. Table 3-XV shows the age of onset of menses of the girls divided by race and amount of body fat. Early maturation in itself may be a deciding factor in obesity development. However, the Negro girls tend to be both

TABLE 3–XIV

PERCENTAGE OF EACH RACIAL GROUP FALLING INTO EACH BODY FAT CLASS

	Boys			Girls		
	CAUCASIAN	NEGRO	ORIENTAL	CAUCASIAN	NEGRO	ORIENTAL
Ninth Grade						
Lean	10.86	8.03	11.63	10.76	4.76	21.43
Somewhat lean	15.36	11.68	25.58	14.87	12.24	23.81
Average	47.57	53.28	53.49	51.58	52.38	30.95
Somewhat obese	16.10	17.52	0.00	13.29	16.33	21.43
Obese	10.11	9.49	9.30	9.49	14.29	2.38
Tenth Grade						
Lean	10.08	7.89	16.67	11.19	3.52	20.59
Somewhat lean	15.50	11.84	22.22	14.55	15.49	17.65
Average	51.55	48.68	50.00	52.61	48.59	32.35
Somewhat obese	13.95	19.74	5.56	14.18	14.79	26.47
Obese	8.91	11.84	5.56	7.46	17.61	2.94
Eleventh Grade						
Lean	11.20	4.76	27.03	10.16	3.60	30.56
Somewhat lean	17.60	10.71	18.92	17.48	12.23	11.11
Average	51.20	50.60	35.14	51.21	51.80	33.33
Somewhat obese	10.00	22.62	13.51	11.79	18.71	22.22
Obese	10.00	11.31	5.41	9.35	13.67	2.78
Twelfth Grade						
Lean	10.27	8.57	14.29	11.02	3.42	21.62
Somewhat lean	17.41	9.29	14.29	17.55	8.55	16.22
Average	49.11	52.14	54.29	51.84	50.43	40.54
Somewhat obese	12.95	18.57	11.43	13.06	17.95	18.92
Obese	10.27	11.43	5.71	6.53	19.66	2.70

TABLE 3–XV

AGE OF ONSET OF MENSES

I. Percent Body Fat Classification (12th grade fat classes)

	X	σ	N
Lean	12.9 *	1.047	35
Somewhat lean	12.7	0.921	48
Average	12.5	1.101	175
Somewhat obese	12.6	1.291	54
Obese	12.2 *	1.236	29

II. Race Classification

	X	σ	N
Caucasian	12.7 *	1.180	240
Negro	12.3 *	1.169	137
Oriental	12.7	0.856	36

* Statistically significant differences (0.05 level).

fatter (Table 3-XIV) and earlier maturers (Table 3-XV) than the Caucasian girls while the Oriental girls tend to be leaner but not later maturers than the Caucasian girls. Since the lean girls, regardless of race, mature later than other girls, we might assume that body composition is more strongly related to age of maturation than it is to ethnic origin. If this is true and if menarchal age is an inherited trait as Tanner (1966) has said seems probable, then it may follow that the tendency to become obese also is an inherited trait.

Another comparison that may indicate that heredity plays a role in the development of obesity is that between body composition of parents and that of children. (In comparing children and parents we cannot, however, rule out environmental factors.)

We invited the parents of the subjects in our substudy to come to our offices to be measured. Unfortunately, we had few volunteers. As shown in Table 3-XVI, the trends indicate that parents of lean children tend to be leaner than other parents. This tendency seems to be most pronounced for the mothers of girls. This is in line with the observation of Withers (1964) that mothers contribute ectomorphy or endomorphy to their offspring while fathers contribute mesomorphy.

The data reported in Tables 3-XVII, 3-XVIII, and 3-XIX, though including more subjects, are open to some question. These data were gathered by mailed questionnaires inquiring about height and weight of mother and father. We used the heights and weights from these responses to assign the parents to overweight categories. The standards we used were based on "Desirable Weights for Men and Women according to Height and Frame" (Metropolitan Life Insurance Company, Nov.–Dec., 1959). We used the highest weight for the large frame size for each height as a reference point in assigning parents to the overweight categories. By this method, we might have classified as normal many parents who were actually overweight; but few whom we classified as overweight were likely to be nonobese.

Table 3-XVII indicates that about 17 percent of the mothers and 9 percent of the fathers were overweight. However, almost 45 percent of the mothers of obese boys and girls were overweight and about 20 percent of the fathers of obese boys and girls were overweight. Thirteen percent of all the parents were overweight. However, 33 percent of those with obese children were overweight and 17 percent of those with somewhat obese children were overweight.

There seemed to be little difference in the trends between parents and sex of child except that more mothers of girls were

TABLE 3-XVI

MEAN PER CENT BODY FAT OF FATHERS AND MOTHERS CLASSIFIED BY SEX AND FAT CLASS OF CHILD

Fat Class of Child	FATHERS					MOTHERS				
	Boys	N	Girls	N	$\bar{X}$ of Fathers	Boys	N	Girls	N	$\bar{X}$ of Mothers
Lean	15.14	5	10.75	8	12.44	18.35	7	13.98	11	15.68
Somewhat lean	14.35	5	17.61	3	15.57	21.11	7	16.39	5	19.14
Average	18.43	16	14.19	18	16.19	18.07	17	19.46	23	18.87
Somewhat obese	17.32	4	21.82	4	19.57	18.04	7	28.14	4	21.71
Obese	21.58	4	—	0	21.58	21.72	6	29.74	2	23.72
All	17.59	34	14.59	33	16.11	19.59	44	19.01	45	19.04

TABLE 3–XVII

PERCENTAGE OF OVERWEIGHT PARENTS OF BOYS AND GIRLS CLASSIFIED BY TWELFTH-GRADE FAT CLASS OF CHILD

Boys and Girls 12th Grade Body Fat Class	Mothers			Fathers			Total Parents		
	Total N	10–20% overweight %	20% plus overweight %	Total N	10–20% overweight %	20% plus overweight %	Total N	10–20% overweight %	20% plus overweight %
Lean	53	5.66	7.55	54	7.41	0.00	107	6.54	3.74
Somewhat lean	79	5.06	3.80	74	0.00	2.70	153	2.61	3.27
Average	272	6.99	6.62	263	6.08	1.90	535	6.54	4.30
Somewhat obese	65	7.69	12.31	62	8.06	6.45	127	7.87	9.45
Obese	54	16.67	27.78	46	15.22	4.35	100	16.00	17.00
Total Group	523	7.65	9.18	499	6.41	2.61	1022	7.04	5.97

TABLE 3-XVIII

PERCENTAGE OF OVERWEIGHT PARENTS OF GIRLS CLASSIFIED BY TWELFTH-GRADE FAT CLASS OF CHILD

GIRLS	MOTHERS			FATHERS			TOTAL PARENTS		
12th Grade Body Fat Class	Total N	10–20% overweight %	20% plus overweight %	Total N	10–20% overweight %	20% plus overweight %	Total N	10–20% overweight %	20% plus overweight %
Lean	34	5.88	8.82	33	6.06	0.00	67	5.97	4.48
Somewhat lean	38	7.89	2.63	35	0.00	0.00	73	4.11	1.37
Average	132	9.09	7.58	125	3.20	3.20	257	6.23	5.45
Somewhat obese	39	10.26	12.82	37	8.11	8.11	76	9.21	10.53
Obese	23	8.70	39.13	20	15.00	5.00	43	11.63	23.26
Total Groups	266	8.65	10.53	250	4.80	3.20	516	6.78	6.98

TABLE 3-XIX

PERCENTAGE OF OVERWEIGHT PARENTS OF BOYS CLASSIFIED BY TWELFTH-GRADE FAT CLASS OF CHILD

Boys	Mothers			Fathers			Total Parents		
12th Grade Body Fat Class	Total N	10–20% overweight %	20% plus overweight %	Total N	10–20% overweight %	20% plus overweight %	Total N	10–20% overweight %	20% plus overweight %
Lean	19	5.26	5.26	21	9.52	0.00	40	7.50	2.50
Somewhat lean	41	2.44	4.88	39	0.00	5.13	80	1.25	5.00
Average	140	5.00	5.71	138	8.70	0.72	278	6.83	3.24
Somewhat obese	26	3.85	11.54	25	8.00	4.00	51	5.88	7.84
Obese	31	22.58	19.35	26	15.38	3.85	57	19.30	12.28
Total Group	257	6.61	7.78	249	8.03	2.01	506	7.31	4.94

overweight (Table 3-XVIII) than mothers of boys (Table 3-XIX).

Summary

We found that the anthropometric method of determining body composition correlated fairly well with other methods, and that it was practical for use within the schools.

Using arbitrary cut-off points, 10 to 18 percent of these teen-agers were obese, depending on age and sex.

Skeletal growth is apparent in boys and—contrary to popular conceptions—girls, throughout the high school years, with that of the boys more rapid. Boys and girls also showed increase in muscle mass during this period. The boys increased in body fat significantly only from the eleventh to the twelfth grade, and girls increased in body fat from the tenth to the eleventh grade and decreased from the eleventh to the twelfth grade. The increase for the girls might be a normal development and the subsequent decrease might be a result of voluntary weight reduction.

Significant differences in many measurements between teen-agers of different ethnic origin may indicate that the same standards should not be applied to all races. Negro boys and girls have smaller bi-iliac and bitrochanteric to stature ratios than Oriental or Caucasian boys and girls. Caucasian boys and girls have smaller biacromial to stature ratios than do Oriental or Negro boys and girls. Oriental boys and girls tend to have larger diameter to stature ratios than do the other boys and girls. These differences in body conformation make it desirable to separate the ethnic groups when comparing typical anthropometric measurements that might characterize the lean or obese. Negro boys and girls tend to have a greater percentage of body fat than do Caucasian or Oriental boys and girls. The tendency for the obese group of girls to have larger diameter to stature ratios is more pronounced in Caucasian girls than it is in any other racial group of girls or in any racial group of boys.

Certain tendencies appear in the whole sample, however. Obese boys are taller than other boys, especially in the ninth grade; this difference tends to disappear by the twelfth grade.

Lean girls tend to be taller than the other girls in the ninth through the twelfth grades. The bitrochanteric to stature ratio is the one index that is most likely to be larger for the obese groups for both sexes and three races. While obese boys and girls tend to have broader bone structure in relation to height than do other groups, the predictive value of broad bone structure in anticipating future obesity seems to be fairly good for boys and poor for girls.

The observed differences (genetic, environmental, and ethnic) and their relationship to the development of obesity should be further investigated in order to better identify those groups or individuals who may be potentially obese. Programs for obesity control could then be specifically designed to help these groups or individuals.

CHAPTER 4

CALORIC AND NUTRIENT INTAKES
AND EATING PRACTICES*

A S PREVIOUSLY INDICATED, a subsample of subjects was chosen on the basis of body composition for study of food intake and activity. Subjects were asked at four different times throughout the four years of the study to record what they ate and how much time they spent in various activities for a seven-day period.

The number of subjects completing diet and activity records decreased from an initial group of 184 to 127 who kept records during the fourth weekly period; only 122 subjects completed all four weeks. (See Chapter 2 for procedure.) Those who completed all four weeks will be referred to as the longitudinal subsample. We found that the obese subjects were less inclined to complete all four records than other subjects.

Caloric and Nutrient Intakes

Mean caloric and nutrient values from all dietary records completed during the four weekly periods are indicated as per cent of the 1964 Recommended Dietary Allowances (Food and Nutrition Board, 1964) for teenagers (ages 16 years to 17.5 years) in Figure 4–1. With the exception of girls' calcium and iron intakes, these values seem satisfactory. However, when subjects were classified by their intake level of some nutrients as in Table 4-I, the picture was not as bright. In addition to low intakes of calcium and iron, low levels of ascorbic acid, vitamin A and, in boys, thiamine also appear in a relatively large proportion

---

* A portion of this chapter appeared originally in the *Journal of the American Dietetic Association*, 50:385, May 1967 and 53:17, July 1968. We are indebted to the publication for the use of the material.

of subjects. On the other hand, an even greater percentage exceeded the recommended allowances for these same nutrients. In virtually no subjects did low intakes of protein or niacin occur.

We compared the values shown in Figure 4–1 with the mean nutrient intakes for four weeks of only those subjects who completed all four weeks' records. The values are slightly higher in the four weeks' mean for the longitudinal sample than shown in Figure 4–1 but the differences are very small. However, when the percentages of subjects having low mean nutrient intakes for four weeks (longitudinal sample, Table 4-I) were compared with those for the total sample's mean intake for one week, we found some differences: Fifteen percent of the girls in the longitudinal sample had intakes of ascorbic acid below two thirds of the Recommended Dietary Allowances for four weekly periods; 30 percent of the girls in the total sample had intakes below this level on a weekly basis; 20 percent of the boys in the longitudinal sample had intakes of calcium below two thirds of the Recommended Dietary Allowances for four weekly periods; and 30 percent of all the boys had intakes below this level on a weekly basis. The rest of the percentages were approximately the same.

The percentage of subjects having nutrient intakes below two thirds of the Recommended Dietary Allowances, as well as the mean nutrient intakes, indicates that the most neglected nutrients for the girls are iron and calcium, and ascorbic acid and calcium for the boys.

When one considers the somewhat high Recommended Dietary Allowance for iron and the food sources available, it is perhaps understandable that so many girls on a fairly low level of caloric consumption failed to meet two thirds of the Recommended Dietary Allowance of this mineral. However, there seems to be no reason for the girls or boys to have diets low in calcium if they have the "milk-drinking" habit.

While the protein intakes of our subjects were fairly high, they were not nearly as high as those of the Iowa teenagers reported by Hodges and Krehl (1965). The boys of the Iowa study reported caloric intakes of about 3,500 while the mean caloric intake of our boys was considerably lower—about 2,800. The Iowa girls averaged about 2,450 calories per day while our girls aver-

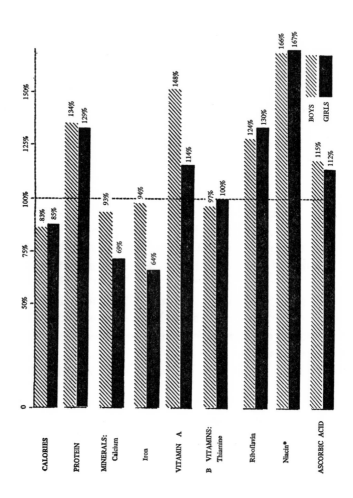

Figure 4–1. Mean caloric and nutrient intake as per cent of recommended dietary allowance—four seven-day records, total subsample. Milligram equivalents of niacin were calculated as 1 per cent of protein intake as tryptophan and a conversion factor of 60 mg to 1 mg niacin (Horwitt, 1958) was used.

aged a little less than 2,000 calories per day. (It should be pointed out that the Iowa results are based on dietary histories rather than records.) Because of the lower caloric levels, the lower protein levels of our subjects represented a larger protein contribution to the caloric intake. The Iowa teenagers had about 12 percent of the calories from protein and our subjects averaged about 16 percent. Our subjects appeared to have heights comparable to the Iowa subjects of about the same age, and our girls appeared to be of about the same weight. The Iowa boys, however, appeared to weigh more at each year than did our boys.

Even though the results of each week of the dietary records were similar, there was a tendency for both boys and girls to con-

TABLE 4–I

PERCENT OF SUBJECTS HAVING VARIOUS LEVELS OF CALORIC AND NUTRIENT INTAKES AS MEASURED BY RECOMMENDED DIETARY ALLOWANCES—MEAN VALUES FROM FOUR SEVEN-DAY RECORDS, LONGITUDINAL SUBSAMPLE

	Recommended Dietary Allowances—Plus		Two-thirds Recommended Dietary Allowances To Recommended Dietary Allowances		Below Two-thirds Recommended Dietary Allowances	
	%	N	%	N	%	N
			BOYS N = 51			
Calories	17.65	9	64.71	33	17.65	9
Protein	86.27	44	9.80	5	3.92	2
Calcium	41.18	21	39.22	20	19.61	10
Iron	39.22	20	49.02	25	11.76	6
Vitamin A	70.59	36	19.61	10	9.80	5
Thiamine	43.14	22	43.14	22	13.73	7
Riboflavin	78.43	40	17.65	9	3.92	2
Niacin *	94.12	48	5.88	3	0.00	0
Ascorbic acid	49.02	25	19.61	10	31.37	16
			GIRLS N = 71			
	%	N	%	N	%	N
Calories	18.31	13	66.20	47	15.49	11
Protein	87.32	62	12.68	9	0.00	0
Calcium	12.68	9	38.03	27	49.30	35
Iron	0.00	0	42.25	30	57.75	41
Vitamin A	49.30	35	35.21	25	15.49	11
Thiamine	46.48	33	47.89	34	5.63	4
Riboflavin	83.10	59	12.68	9	4.23	3
Niacin *	100.00	71	0.00	0	0.00	0
Ascorbic acid	49.30	35	35.21	25	15.49	11

* Milligram equivalents of niacin were calculated as one percent of protein intake as tryptophan and a conversion factor of 60 mg dietary tryptophan equivalent to 1 mg niacin (Horwitt, 1958) was used.

sume more calories as well as higher levels of calcium, thiamine, riboflavin, and ascorbic acid during the school year than during vacation (Table 4-II). These differences are not statistically significant except for the girls' intake of calcium, which was higher in spring, 1965, than in summer, 1963, or summer, 1964. They may reflect a trend toward more regular eating as well as general living habits during the school year. These differences among the four records prompted us to report the mean of these records for the longitudinal sample to give a more nearly complete picture of the dietary intakes of this group.

We will report in detail only the first week's records which were completed by the largest number of subjects and the mean of all four weeks completed by the longitudinal sample.

Seven-day Dietary Records

Table 4-III shows the mean caloric and nutrient intakes of boys and girls classified according to amount of body fat, race, and socioeconomic level. These intakes are for one week in the summer of 1963 when subjects were approximately sixteen years old. Mean caloric and nutrient intakes are significantly lower for girls than boys (0.05 level) except vitamin A, ascorbic acid, and per cent of calories from fat, carbohydrate, and protein. Although the difference is not significant, the boys had a slightly larger percentage of their caloric intake from fat than did the girls.

BODY FAT CLASS. The intake of calories of the average boys is significantly higher than that of all other male fat classes. Correspondingly, nutrient intakes of the average boys were higher than those of some of the other male fat classes. There are no differences between the groups in the percentage of calories from fat and protein. For the girls, the higher caloric intake of the lean group is significantly different from average, somewhat obese, and obese groups of girls. While there are some significant differences in levels of nutrient intake among the girls, the actual values are such that the statistical tests may not represent really practical nutritional differences. The mean values of the boys are all above two-thirds of the Recommended Dietary Allowances. The mean values of calcium and iron for the girls are below two-thirds of the same allowances for all except the lean group.

TABLE 4-IIA

MEAN CALORIC AND NUTRIENT INTAKE FROM EACH OF FOUR SEVEN-DAY RECORDS—TOTAL SUBSAMPLE

BOYS

NUTRIENTS	Summer 1963 N = 90		Spring 1964 N = 73		Summer 1964 N = 62		Spring 1965 N = 54	
	X̄	σ	X̄	σ	X̄	σ	X̄	σ
Calories	2796	772.0	2908	766.1	2732	807.9	2833	845.7
Protein (gm)	112	37.0	116	31.9	112	37.4	117	41.5
Fat (gm)	132	42.3	142	46.3	130	47.2	133	41.5
Carbohydrate (gm)	305	94.9	305	87.1	289	97.2	304	102.9
% Calories from fat	42.0	5.74	43.7	5.48	42.6	6.92	42.3	5.00
% Calories from protein	16.0	2.68	16.0	2.17	16.4	2.78	16.6	2.94
% Calories from carbohydrate *	42.0		40.3		41.0		41.1	
Calcium (mg)	1264	574.1	1360	520.6	1196	552.3	1406	653.9
Iron (mg)	14.1	4.26	14.3	4.38	14.1	5.39	13.9	4.95
Vitamin A (IU)	6743	4096	7905	6732	8087	9632	6924	5876
Thiamine (mg)	1.35	0.423	1.38	0.454	1.31	0.485	1.38	0.546
Riboflavin (mg)	2.41	0.924	2.56	0.856	2.34	0.947	2.62	1.129
Niacin (mg)	19.3	6.23	19.6	5.85	19.4	6.46	19.9	7.10
Ascorbic acid (mg)	81	56.4	91	63.1	89	68.0	108	121.1

* Calculated by difference.

TABLE 4–IIB

GIRLS

Nutrients	Summer 1963 N = 94		Spring 1964 N = 86		Summer 1964 N = 82		Spring 1965 N = 73	
	X	σ	X	σ	X	σ	X	σ
Calories	1960	506.7	2000	495.0	1876	520.3	1959	497.5
Protein (gm)	73	18.7	75	19.6	74	21.1	79	21.5
Fat (gm)	89	28.3	92	28.3	84	27.3	88	27.0
Carbohydrate (gm)	228	63.0	229	57.1	217	65.8	223	63.7
% Calories from fat	40.7	5.06	41.0	5.00	39.9	5.75	40.3	6.02
% Calories from protein	15.0	2.30	15.2	2.23	16.1	3.05	16.2	2.86
% Calories from carbohydrate *	44.3		43.8		44.0		43.5	
Calcium (mg)	857	322.0	906	345.3	833	409.8	993	478.6
Iron (mg)	9.7	2.35	9.6	2.16	9.4	2.42	9.5	2.48
Vitamin A (IU)	6254	4258	5562	3405	6170	4637	4766	3194
Thiamine (mg)	0.90	0.266	0.92	0.242	0.88	0.266	0.90	0.240
Riboflavin (mg)	1.66	0.521	1.71	0.530	1.63	0.626	1.77	0.689
Niacin (mg)	12.9	3.53	12.7	3.31	13.1	3.90	13.2	3.74
Ascorbic acid (mg)	75	43.9	86	52.3	73	40.6	82	51.2

* Calculated by difference.

TABLE 4-IIIA

MEAN CALORIC AND NUTRIENT INTAKE FROM SEVEN-DAY RECORDS, SUMMER 1963
SUBJECTS CLASSIFIED BY PERCENT BODY FAT, RACE, AND SOCIOECONOMIC LEVEL—BOYS

NUTRIENTS		Fat Class					Race			Socioeconomic Level †		
		Lean 14	Somewhat Lean 16	Average 30	Somewhat Obese 8	Obese 22	Caucasian 54	Negro 24	Oriental 12	Lower Third 8	Middle Third 52	Upper Third 30
Calories	X̄	2595	2463	3178	2808	2641	2889	2625	2687	2205	2823	2895
	σ	572.9	545.8	945.1	486.5	672.6	826.0	669.0	650.0	625.2	670.0	903.2
Protein (gm)	X̄	101	94	133	115	101	116	96	122	89	112	116
	σ	29.5	24.8	44.4	30.3	29.0	37.6	31.1	37.7	42.3	33.4	40.0
Fat (gm)	X̄	122	114	148	133	125	136	120	130	97	134	134
	σ	32.6	34.2	52.4	33.2	34.4	41.9	39.8	43.6	43.5	36.8	46.3
Carbohydrate (gm)	X̄	286	276	344	299	289	316	299	270	254	304	323
	σ	70.0	69.5	113.2	49.6	99.1	103.8	86.9	53.3	53.3	91.2	105.7
% Calories from fat	X̄	42.2	41.4	41.5	42.4	42.8	42.4	40.8	42.7	38.0	42.8	41.6
	σ	4.88	6.60	6.10	4.80	5.73	5.07	6.74	6.52	8.14	5.63	4.81
% Calories from protein	X̄	15.5	15.3	16.8	16.2	15.5	16.1	14.6	18.1	15.6	15.9	16.1
	σ	2.88	2.32	2.62	2.53	2.88	2.46	2.47	2.65	4.13	2.78	1.94
% Calories from carbohydrate *	X̄	42.3	43.3	41.7	41.4	41.7	41.5	44.6	39.2	46.4	41.3	42.3
Calcium (mg)	X̄	1303	989	1504	1318	1076	1422	973	1106	879	1177	1506
	σ	496.0	466.7	697.0	516.3	373.8	603.7	401.3	467.9	372.1	470.0	682.4
Iron (mg)	X̄	12.2	12.0	16.3	14.4	13.6	14.2	13.2	14.5	12.2	14.4	13.8
	σ	2.87	2.43	5.27	3.57	3.39	4.33	3.89	3.48	5.24	3.52	4.67
Vitamin A (IU)	X̄	5500	5400	8400	5500	6600	7518	4675	7308	4175	6538	7750
	σ	2640	2470	4980	3630	4070	3817	3147	5579	1058	4158	4179
Thiamine (mg)	X̄	1.31	1.07	1.54	1.45	1.27	1.40	1.27	1.24	1.05	1.37	1.38
	σ	0.487	0.264	0.479	0.326	0.300	0.462	0.349	0.343	0.373	0.367	0.499
Riboflavin (mg)	X̄	2.31	1.92	2.87	2.53	2.16	2.60	1.98	2.32	1.74	2.35	2.65
	σ	0.748	0.750	1.135	0.740	0.593	0.935	0.682	0.962	0.732	0.790	1.062
Niacin (mg)	X̄	16.4	16.2	22.9	18.9	18.8	19.6	17.4	21.5	17.5	20.0	18.5
	σ	4.77	3.66	7.02	5.83	5.48	6.36	5.59	6.17	8.54	5.93	6.03
Ascorbic acid (mg)	X̄	70	72	105	74	65	97	52	73	57	71	107
	σ	42.1	37.4	78.8	54.7	24.3	63.6	32.9	32.1	16.5	42.4	74.6

TABLE 4—IIIB—GIRLS

NUTRIENTS	N	Fat Class					Race			Socioeconomic Level †		
		Lean 25	Somewhat Lean 18	Average 36	Somewhat Obese 8	Obese 7	Caucasian 60	Negro 25	Oriental 9	Lower Third 50	Middle Third 50	Upper Third 35
Calories	X̄	2156	2000	1890	1763	1752	1996	1923	1833	1675	1965	2029
	σ	484.3	284.6	563.6	268.0	760.9	516.8	513.6	437.5	312.1	491.5	552.1
Protein (gm)	X̄	82	71	70	66	70	75	65	80	56	73	76
	σ	18.9	11.8	18.7	15.8	26.2	17.8	19.0	18.4	8.0	18.4	19.0
Fat (gm)	X̄	97	90	88	75	82	92	86	77	74	90	92
	σ	25.8	15.4	33.9	22.4	36.2	29.9	25.3	24.1	8.7	28.0	31.4
Carbohydrate (gm)	X̄	250	239	217	216	193	229	231	213	204	226	236
	σ	58.4	50.4	67.1	36.9	91.0	63.8	67.8	45.8	64.7	61.6	64.6
% Calories from fat	X̄	40.3	40.7	41.3	37.9	42.1	41.3	40.4	37.7	40.6	40.9	40.3
	σ	3.96	4.87	5.78	6.82	2.01	5.27	4.69	3.83	4.66	5.66	4.32
% Calories from protein	X̄	15.5	14.2	15.0	15.1	16.3	15.3	13.5	17.5	13.7	15.1	15.4
	σ	2.38	1.68	2.29	3.50	1.21	2.02	2.03	2.08	2.04	2.25	2.36
% Calories from carbohydrate *	X̄	44.2	45.1	43.7	47.0	41.6	43.4	46.1	44.8	45.7	44.0	44.3
Calcium (mg)	X̄	986	847	830	686	759	926	669	921	539	878	910
	σ	325.9	306.0	319.8	257.8	343.6	294.3	302.4	375.0	124.1	339.0	289.8
Iron (mg)	X̄	10.6	9.3	9.2	9.6	9.7	9.6	9.8	9.3	8.7	8.7	9.7
	σ	2.63	1.47	2.25	1.74	3.71	2.27	2.63	2.24	1.81	2.50	2.25
Vitamin A (IU)	X̄	5600	5600	6900	8500	4400	6625	5576	5667	5233	7054	5374
	σ	2970	2880	5070	6320	3120	4431	3654	4800	4174	5133	2346
Thiamine (mg)	X̄	1.02	0.86	0.88	0.81	0.85	0.92	0.89	0.84	0.75	0.93	0.90
	σ	0.302	0.159	0.263	0.210	0.361	0.250	0.317	0.227	0.178	0.275	0.264
Riboflavin (mg)	X̄	1.83	1.60	1.62	1.64	1.45	1.76	1.39	1.79	1.22	1.73	1.68
	σ	0.522	0.456	0.505	0.603	0.654	0.484	0.524	0.544	0.226	0.553	0.480
Niacin (mg)	X̄	14.1	11.8	12.7	13.1	12.5	12.9	12.5	14.1	11.9	13.2	12.8
	σ	3.57	2.47	3.67	3.24	4.84	3.39	3.58	4.43	3.19	3.78	3.28
Ascorbic acid (mg)	X̄	80	69	80	59	61	83	59	64	54	75	80
	σ	39.1	36.2	47.2	38.1	67.0	43.7	41.3	42.8	30.4	48.9	38.2

* Calculated by difference.
† U.S. Census of Population: 1960, California—Table 76 "Income in 1959 of Families and Persons, and Weeks Worked in 1959 for Standard Metropolitan Statistical Areas, Urbanized Areas, and Urban Places of 10,000 and more; 1960," Urban Places—Berkeley. Lower-third: under $1,000–$5,110; Middle-third: $5,111–$8,586; Upper-third: $8,587 and over.

RACE. Racial classifications show some significant differences. Caucasian boys had higher intakes of protein, calcium, vitamin A, riboflavin, and ascorbic acid than the Negro boys. Oriental boys had higher intakes of protein, vitamin A, niacin, and ascorbic acid than the Negro boys. Caucasian boys had higher intakes of carbohydrate, calcium, and ascorbic acid than the Oriental boys. Negro boys had a mean intake of ascorbic acid barely below two thirds of the Recommended Dietary Allowance. Nutrient intakes of Oriental and Caucasian girls showed no significant differences. Both groups had higher intakes of protein, calcium and riboflavin than the Negro girls. Negro girls had mean intakes of calcium below two thirds of the Recommended Dietary Allowance, and all the girls had mean intakes of iron below two thirds of the Recommended Dietary Allowance.

SOCIOECONOMIC LEVEL. Socioeconomic classifications were defined on the basis of median income of the census tract in which the subjects resided. Mean caloric intakes of the lower-third level of both sexes are significantly lower than the caloric intake of the other two levels. The mean nutrient intakes of the lower socioeconomic level are also significantly lower than those of the other two levels for some, but not all, of the nutrients. The boys in the lower-third level had mean intakes of calories and calcium below two thirds of the Recommended Dietary Allowances. The lower- and middle-third levels of the girls had mean intakes of calcium below two thirds of the Recommended Dietary Allowances. All levels of girls fell below two thirds of the Recommended Dietary Allowance in mean intakes of iron.

Mean Daily Nutrient Intakes from Four Seven-Day Records

Table 4-IV shows the caloric and nutrient intakes for all boys, all girls, and for boys and girls subdivided into groups according to amount of body fat, race, and socioeconomic level. Statistically significant differences again occur between the boys and girls for all intakes except vitamin A, ascorbic acid, and percentage of calories from fat, protein, and carbohydrate. Again, though the difference is not significant, the boys obtained a larger percentage of their calories from fat than the girls.

BODY FAT CLASS. Significant differences for the boys and girls

TABLE 4-IVA

MEAN CALORIC AND NUTRIENT INTAKE FROM FOUR SEVEN-DAY RECORDS, LONGITUDINAL SAMPLE
SUBJECTS CLASSIFIED BY PERCENT BODY FAT, RACE, AND SOCIOECONOMIC LEVEL—BOYS

NUTRIENTS	N	All 51	Fat Class — Lean 9	Somewhat Lean 7	Average 19	Somewhat Obese 7	Obese 7	Race — Caucasian 31	Negro 10	Oriental 10	Socioeconomic Level † — Lower Third 3	Middle Third 27	Upper Third 21
Calories	X̄	2846	2675	2923	3088	2621	2624	3084	2426	2529	2364	2730	3064
	σ	116.2	550.6	1273.5	566.0	779.1	817.1	789.8	754.1	494.4	247.8	673.5	912.4
Protein (gm)	X̄	116	107	130	126	101	107	125	92	114	98	112	125
	σ	37.5	25.7	62.2	26.6	38.4	31.4	38.8	33.3	24.8	20.4	32.2	43.5
Fat (gm)	X̄	135	130	144	144	121	127	145	116	121	121	129	144
	σ	42.1	35.0	62.4	33.8	43.4	39.1	41.7	43.8	30.0	23.8	38.3	47.1
Carbohydrate (gm)	X̄	305	284	293	337	296	273	337	263	251	232	291	335
	σ	96.7	77.2	133.3	83.0	89.2	102.9	97.4	89.4	53.2	55.9	81.5	109.5
% Calories from fat	X̄	42.5	43.4	44.3	41.7	40.8	43.9	42.4	42.5	42.9	46.0	42.4	42.2
	σ	5.66	6.55	4.15	5.05	7.01	4.66	5.02	7.84	5.08	6.96	5.61	5.44
% Calories from protein	X̄	16.3	16.1	17.7	16.4	15.2	16.5	16.2	15.1	18.1	16.5	16.3	16.3
	σ	2.67	2.43	2.49	2.70	2.81	2.31	2.54	2.64	2.23	3.32	2.80	2.42
% Calories from carbohydrates *	X̄	41.2	40.5	38.0	41.9	44.0	39.6	41.4	42.4	39.0	37.5	41.3	41.5
Calcium (mg)	X̄	1338	1201	1538	1461	1193	1162	1519	965	1148	1078	1249	1489
	σ	575.0	427.9	914.5	475.5	571.9	436.8	606.4	420.4	316.8	268.7	495.6	662.6
Iron (mg)	X̄	14.3	12.9	15.7	15.6	12.7	13.2	15.3	12.0	13.3	11.8	13.6	15.4
	σ	4.86	3.28	8.91	3.62	4.02	3.66	5.23	4.06	3.19	2.36	3.66	6.11
Vitamin A (IU)	X̄	7493	7247	9546	8236	5889	5800	8744	3945	7160	7117	6790	8450
	σ	7007	6671	13774	5139	3394	4583	8056	1892	5413	6035	5597	8560
Thiamine (mg)	X̄	1.38	1.24	1.47	1.52	1.27	1.23	1.49	1.18	1.23	1.11	1.34	1.47
	σ	0.492	0.339	0.852	0.377	0.437	0.418	0.522	0.413	0.359	0.288	0.385	0.608
Riboflavin (mg)	X̄	2.53	2.35	2.85	2.76	2.21	2.25	2.79	1.92	2.32	2.17	2.43	2.71
	σ	0.980	0.838	1.561	0.782	0.881	0.809	1.046	0.697	0.647	0.695	0.877	1.109
Niacin (mg)	X̄	19.7	18.5	20.6	21.0	17.8	19.2	20.8	16.4	19.6	17.6	19.2	20.6
	σ	6.30	4.95	9.95	4.72	5.49	7.32	6.46	5.81	5.11	4.53	5.65	7.17
Ascorbic acid (mg)	X̄	94	78	125	107	86	62	118	43	73	61	77	122
	σ	83.2	47.7	162.3	72.3	47.8	48.7	95.9	26.8	37.6	23.6	53.6	108.8

TABLE 4-IVB—GIRLS

			Fat Class					Race			Socioeconomic Level †		
NUTRIENTS	N	All 71	Lean 14	Somewhat Lean 10	Average 31	Somewhat Obese 10	Obese 6	Caucasian 45	Negro 17	Oriental 9	Lower Third 6	Middle Third 39	Upper Third 26
Calories	X̄	1972	2112	2102	1981	1771	1717	1982	1972	1920	1776	2018	1949
	σ	486.6	431.3	356.7	496.9	444.7	618.2	512.1	479.2	361.6	381.1	499.9	479.1
Protein (gm)	X̄	76	85	83	74	70	68	78	69	81	64	77	77
	σ	19.9	19.2	17.5	19.1	17.7	23.6	20.2	18.5	17.4	13.4	20.5	19.3
Fat (gm)	X̄	89	99	94	89	78	78	90	90	83	80	92	87
	σ	27.0	26.3	22.5	27.7	23.1	29.0	28.3	25.5	22.5	19.0	28.1	26.5
Carbohydrate (gm)	X̄	227	233	243	233	207	194	227	231	221	209	232	225
	σ	61.1	51.9	45.8	62.3	59.9	81.3	65.4	58.9	40.0	57.2	62.2	60.0
% Calories from fat	X̄	40.4	41.8	40.1	40.0	39.6	41.2	40.5	40.9	38.8	40.7	40.7	39.8
	σ	5.43	5.18	4.52	5.62	5.70	5.62	5.96	4.07	4.62	3.87	5.64	5.40
% Calories from protein	X̄	15.6	16.1	16.1	15.0	16.1	16.1	16.0	14.1	16.9	14.6	15.5	16.0
	σ	2.56	2.42	2.94	2.39	2.54	2.63	2.47	2.26	2.20	2.34	2.60	2.49
% Calories from carbohydrates *	X̄	44.0	42.1	43.8	45.0	44.3	42.7	43.5	45.0	44.3	44.7	43.8	44.2
Calcium (mg)	X̄	917	1021	1022	887	845	784	989	708	957	595	929	975
	σ	400.9	415.5	305.0	388.2	406.7	492.6	409.7	317.5	367.1	229.1	415.8	376.6
Iron (mg)	X̄	9.6	10.1	10.4	9.4	9.1	9.0	9.5	9.8	9.8	9.6	9.9	9.2
	σ	2.30	2.15	2.15	2.24	1.97	3.13	2.44	2.17	1.74	2.22	2.31	2.24
Vitamin A (IU)	X̄	5637	4896	6785	5552	5465	6175	5513	6216	5161	6604	6165	4621
	σ	4022	2228	4942	4098	4417	4334	3788	4993	2947	4820	4737	1948
Thiamine (mg)	X̄	0.91	1.00	0.98	0.88	0.89	0.85	0.92	0.90	0.91	0.91	0.94	0.88
	σ	0.251	0.222	0.277	0.223	0.275	0.311	0.270	0.228	0.199	0.189	0.268	0.235
Riboflavin (mg)	X̄	1.72	1.86	1.88	1.66	1.63	1.56	1.79	1.51	1.73	1.34	1.77	1.72
	σ	0.601	0.601	0.456	0.589	0.591	0.795	0.605	0.584	0.533	0.478	0.625	0.563
Niacin (mg)	X̄	13.1	14.2	14.3	12.6	12.6	12.4	13.0	13.4	13.2	13.0	13.5	12.6
	σ	3.52	3.17	2.85	3.56	3.29	4.64	3.61	3.50	3.23	3.27	3.62	3.40
Ascorbic acid (mg)	X̄	82	89	99	75	82	69	91	61	75	78	81	84
	σ	48.2	42.9	51.6	47.3	50.7	47.6	51.0	38.2	37.6	42.9	52.0	43.5

* Calculated by difference.
† U.S. Census of Population: 1960, California—Table 76 "Income in 1959 of Families and Persons, and Weeks Worked in 1959 for Standard Metropolitan Statistical Areas, Urbanized Areas, and Urban Places of 10,000 and more; 1960," Urban Places—Berkeley. Lower-third: under $1,000–$5,110; Middle-third: $5,111–$8,586; Upper-third: $8,587 and over.

in different body fat classes similar to those in the single seven-day records are apparent (Table 4-III). The lean girls and average boys consumed more calories than the other groups. The facts that the obese boys had a significantly lower caloric intake than the average boys and that the obese girls had lower caloric intakes than lean girls are comparable to findings of others (Johnson, Burke and Mayer, 1956; Morgan, 1959; Stefanik, Heald and Mayer, 1959) that the obese consume fewer rather than more calories than their nonobese peers. Hodges and Krehl (1965), however, found that higher body weight corresponded with higher caloric intake.

Our observed lower caloric intake for the obese groups may be due to several factors. Beaudoin and Mayer (1953) found that obese women tended to underestimate their food intake when keeping records. Similarly, the obese teenagers may well have been psychologically motivated to eat less than usual during record-keeping periods.

RACE. Differences between races show statistical significance similar to those described for the seven-day records. As found in the seven-day records, the Negro boys had a mean intake of ascorbic acid below two thirds of the Recommended Dietary Allowance, and the Negro girls had a mean intake of calcium below two thirds of the Recommended Dietary Allowance.

SOCIOECONOMIC LEVEL. Significant differences are also similar to those of the seven-day records in that those girls in the lower third had a mean intake of calcium below two thirds of the Recommended Dietary Allowance.

[Determination of the significance of differences between nutrient means was complicated by the small size of the samples and the significance of differences between standard deviations. A suitable statistical method was found and used which met these limitations (Scheffe, 1943).]

Caloric Intake as Related to Body Weight, Height, and Lean Body Weight

Since there has long been discussion in the literature (Heald, Daugela and Brunschuyler, 1963) about the best way to measure caloric needs for teenagers, we thought it might shed some light on the matter to measure the recorded caloric intake of our sub-

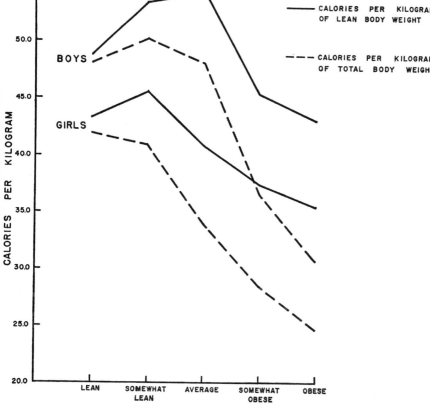

Figure 4–2. Caloric intake per kilogram of body weight and lean body weight—subjects classified by amount of body fat.

jects by several indices. We calculated the calories consumed by each individual as a function of total body weight, lean body weight, and height.

Figure 4–2 shows the results of the mean of the four weeks' intake of calories for the longitudinal sample grouped according to their amount of body fat as a function of weight and lean body weight. There are smaller differences in the groups in calories per kilogram of lean body weight than in calories per kilogram of total body weight. This, of course, may be a reflection of the greater variability of body weight than of lean body weight. Figure 4–2 further emphasizes the lower caloric consumption

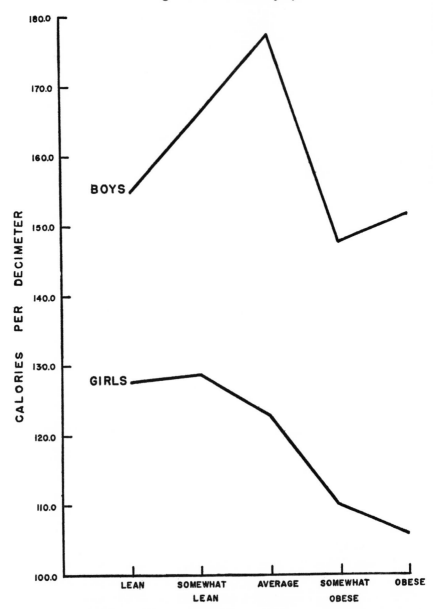

Figure 4–3. Caloric intake per decimeter of height—subjects classified by amount of body fat.

of the obese and somewhat obese subjects as compared with the other groups.

Figure 4–3 showing the caloric consumption per decimeter of height, also reflects the lower mean values of total caloric consumption of the obese boys and girls as shown in Tables 4-III and 4-IV.

We found that for both sexes the caloric intake did not correlate with height, lean body weight, or total body weight.

Eating Practices

Eating Frequency

Table 4-V shows the average number of times food was consumed by the subjects keeping dietary records. There seemed to be a trend toward less frequent eating by the obese subjects of both sexes than those of other fat classifications. The girls appeared to have a slight tendency to eat more frequently than boys. These figures support the popular conception of the teenager as a snacker. We found, generally speaking, that there seemed to be no relationship between the frequency of eating and overall quality of the diet except that those eating less than three times a day usually had much poorer diets. The youngsters who ate frequently were inclined to have overall good diets. It would seem that the snacking habit in the teenage group should not be maligned.

Variability of Intake

Caloric intake as well as intake of nutrients varied greatly from individual to individual and from day to day for each individual. The variation among individuals is emphasized by the large standard deviations shown in Tables 4-III and 4-IV.

In the summer of 1963, the seven-day records of the boys showed an average difference of 2,200 calories between the day on which the most calories were consumed and the day of the least calories. The range of these differences was from 635 calories for the boy with least variation to 4,700 calories for the boy with the greatest variation. For the girls, the average difference was 1,700 calories, with a range from 650 to 6,000

TABLE 4-V

MEAN NUMBER OF TIMES FOOD WAS CONSUMED DURING PERIODS OF DIETARY RECORD-KEEPING—
SUBJECTS CLASSIFIED BY PERCENT BODY FAT

FAT CLASSES	Summer 1963			Spring 1964			Summer 1964			Spring 1965		
	N	Times/Week	Times/Day	N	Times/Week	Times/Day	N	Times/Week	Times/Day	N	Times/Week	Times/Day
Boys												
Lean	14	24.71	3.53	14	27.14	3.88	11	27.45	3.92	12	26.25	3.75
Somewhat lean	16	28.94	4.13	9	24.00	3.43	7	23.14	3.31	7	27.29	3.90
Average	30	27.17	3.88	29	27.03	3.86	23	27.61	3.94	19	27.53	3.93
Somewhat obese	8	28.00	4.00	4	29.50	4.21	10	27.50	3.93	9	27.22	3.89
Obese	22	26.14	3.73	17	22.29	3.18	10	25.20	3.60	7	22.86	3.27
Girls												
Lean	25	28.96	4.14	17	25.88	3.70	15	27.29	3.61	15	28.67	4.10
Somewhat lean	18	31.67	4.52	16	30.81	4.40	11	32.36	4.62	10	30.20	4.31
Average	36	28.94	4.13	35	29.17	4.17	38	28.82	4.12	32	29.78	4.25
Somewhat obese	8	31.38	4.48	11	28.64	4.09	11	25.63	3.66	10	26.70	3.81
Obese	7	24.43	3.49	7	21.57	3.08	7	20.71	2.96	6	21.00	3.00

calories. For the longitudinal sample, we compared the weekly average caloric intake per subject from week to week and found smaller differences. Average daily intakes for the boys showed a difference of 890 calories from the week in which the fewest calories were consumed to the week in which the most calories were consumed, with a range of differences from 260 to 1,750 calories. The girls had an average of 700 calories difference on a weekly basis, with a range of 78 to 2,106 calories. The larger variation in intake from day to day indicates that our subjects ate more variably within the short term of a week than from week to week.

Subjects' Comments Compared With Dietary Records

A series of four questionnaires was administered to the entire study population, one each year, from the ninth to twelfth grades as described in Chapter 2. Daily mean intake of those completing all four weeks of dietary records was compared with some of the answers from the questionnaires. In answer to the question "How do you grade the healthfulness of what you eat?" asked in the ninth and twelfth grades, the small sample of subjects who had completed the four weeks of dietary records and also answered both questionnaires responded about the same as the total sample. Roughly 50 percent responded "good," another 15 to 20 percent "excellent," 25 to 30 percent "fair," and less than 5 percent "poor." There seemed to be little or no relationship between the way the ninth-grade boys graded their own diets and the quality of their diets as judged by the number of nutrients falling below the two-thirds Recommended Dietary Allowances level. However, the ninth- and twelfth-grade girls and twelfth-grade boys who rated their diets as "good" or "excellent" averaged fewer nutrients below the two-thirds Recommended Dietary Allowances level than did those rating their diets "poor" or "fair." Among ninth-grade girls and twelfth-grade boys who rated their diets as "excellent," a larger percentage had diets with all nutrients above the two thirds Recommended Dietary Allowances level than did the groups rating their diets otherwise. Ability to rate their own diets realistically appears in some but not all groups of these teenagers.

The open-ended question "What foods should be eaten every day for health?" was asked in the ninth and eleventh grades. We rated the answers by the number of the "Basic Four" (U.S.D.A., 1958) food groups mentioned. More girls than boys in both grades mentioned the "Basic Four" groups, 50 percent as compared to 30 percent, in both grades. A larger percentage of the boys who mentioned all four of the basic food groups had diets in which no nutrient was below two-thirds of the Recommended Dietary Allowance than did those not mentioning all four. However, of the girls who mentioned all four basic food groups, about the same percentage as those mentioning only three of the four basic food groups had intakes with one or no nutrients below two-thirds of the Recommended Dietary Allowances. Thus, when we use knowledge of the "Basic Four" as a gauge, the finding of others (Hinton *et al.*, 1963; Jalso, Burns and Rivers, 1965) that nutritional knowledge improves food practices agrees with our findings for the boys, but not for the girls.

The answers to the question "How often are you hungry?" did not seem to have any relationship to the frequency of eating. Perhaps the more frequent eaters were not aware of being hungry because they were satisfying this hunger. Also, the term "hungry" can have various interpretations.

School Grades Compared to Diet Records

School grades were supplied to us by the Berkeley Unified School District. We compared those students with grade point averages below and above a "C" grade. There were no differences in the number of nutrients that were below two thirds of the Recommended Dietary Allowances between students with grade averages above and below "C."

Meal Eating and Snacking Patterns *

The common observation that teenagers tend to eat oftener than three times a day has already been documented (Table

---

* Food intake was classified as a "meal" or a "snack" in accordance with the subject's own designation whenever one was given. In other cases, a subjective decision was made by the investigator on the basis of type of food, time of day, and time relation to the previous meal.

4-V). We also showed that obese subjects of both sexes tended to eat less frequently than those of other body fat classifications, and that girls tended to eat more frequently than boys. Table 4-VI, based on the records of only those subjects who kept four food and activity diaries, shows which meals and snacks were eaten most frequently by boys and girls in the various fat classes. The breakfast skippers were indeed the obese boys and girls. The small number of evening snackers reported by this group indicates that bedtime snacking was not replacing breakfast. Somewhat obese and obese boys, however, did report more daytime snacks than other boys. Obese girls, on the other hand, tended to eat fewer snacks and meals than other girls. For both

TABLE 4–VI

AVERAGE NUMBER OF MEALS AND SNACKS PER WEEK
BY SEX AND BODY FAT CLASSES

	N	Breakfast	Lunch	Dinner	Evening Snack	Day Snack	Average Total Eating Times Per Day
Boys							
Lean	(9)	6.0	5.4	6.7	3.2	5.7	3.9
Somewhat lean	(7)	6.0	5.4	7.0	2.9	3.6	3.6
Average	(19)	6.0	5.4	6.8	2.9	6.7	4.0
Somewhat obese	(9)	5.5	5.0	6.4	2.5	7.9	3.9
Obese	(7)	3.9	4.6	6.7	2.6	7.4	3.6
All	(51)	5.6	5.2	6.7	2.9	6.4	3.8
Girls							
Lean	(14)	5.9	5.8	6.6	4.0	6.3	4.1
Somewhat lean	(10)	6.2	5.3	6.4	4.9	9.0	4.5
Average	(31)	5.7	4.9	6.5	4.0	9.1	4.3
Somewhat obese	(10)	6.0	5.4	6.2	2.8	6.4	4.6
Obese	(6)	4.5	4.5	6.0	2.1	4.1	3.0
All	(71)	5.8	5.2	6.4	3.8	7.7	4.1

sexes dinner was the most and lunch the least frequently eaten meal. Lunch was, in fact, omitted more often than breakfast during summer vacations and about equally during the school year. (See Table 4-VII.)

Reasons for skipping lunch varied with the time of year. During the summer vacations, reasons were late breakfasts or lack of planning or provision for lunch. During the school year, the most frequent reason was participation in other activities with or without a snack instead of meal-eating during the lunch period. As shown in Table 4-VII, both boys and girls reported eating breakfast more regularly when they were about sixteen years of age than when they were older.

TABLE 4–VII

AVERAGE NUMBER OF MEALS AND SNACKS PER WEEK
DURING SCHOOL AND VACATION PERIODS

	Summer Vacation 1963	Summer Vacation 1964	School Year Spring 1964	School Year Spring 1965
Approximate age (yrs)	16.0	17.0	16.5	17.5
Boys (N = 51)				
Breakfasts	6.2	5.2	5.7	5.5
Lunches	5.0	4.8	5.6	5.6
Dinners	6.9	6.7	6.8	6.5
Daytime snacks	7.2	6.9	5.6	5.8
Evening snacks	2.9	3.1	2.4	3.0
Girls (N = 71)				
Breakfasts	6.1	5.7	5.6	5.6
Lunches	4.9	4.6	5.7	5.5
Dinners	6.4	6.2	6.6	6.5
Daytime snacks	8.4	8.2	7.3	7.0
Evening snacks	3.8	4.2	3.5	3.7

Table 4-VIII shows the number and percentage of subjects by sex, ethnic origin, and socioeconomic group who had fixed and variable eating patterns. Negro boys and girls tended to eat all meals, especially breakfast and lunch, less regularly than did Caucasians and Orientals. Although Negro and Oriental girls snacked more frequently than Caucasian girls, this was not true for the boys. Caucasian boys were the leading snackers, followed in order by the Negro and Oriental boys.

Meal regularity tended to increase with rise in socioeconomic classification. The boys in the high socioeconomic group snacked the most frequently, and the girls in this group snacked the least often. Both boys and girls in the low socioeconomic group averaged fewer breakfasts and lunches than other boys and girls. However, only a small number of subjects in the low socioeconomic group completed four records.

That the differences between socioeconomic groups are less striking than those between ethnic groups (Table 4-VIII) suggests that an irregular pattern of eating may be more closely associated with ethnic origin than with socioeconomic status.

When meals missed were compared with stated preferences for the various meals, it was found that those who preferred dinner were less likely to skip any meals than those stating

TABLE 4-VIII

REGULARITY OF EATING PATTERNS BY SEX, ETHNIC ORIGIN, AND SOCIOECONOMIC GROUP

| | | All | Ethnic Origin | | | Socioeconomic Group | | |
			Caucasian	Negro	Oriental	Low	Medium	High
Boys	N	51	31	10	10	3	27	21
Regular	N	36.5*	27	1	8.5*	2.0	17.0	17.5
	%	71.6	87.1	10.0	85.0	66.7	63.0	83.3
Irregular	N	14.5*	4	9	1.5*	1.0	10.0	3.5
	%	28.4	12.9	90.0	15.0	33.3	37.0	16.7
Girls	N	71	45	17	9	6	39	26
Regular	N	49	35.5*	5	8.5*	2.0	25.5	21.5
	%	69.0	78.9	29.4	94.4	33.3	65.4	82.7
Irregular	N	22	9.5	12	0.5*	4.0	13.5	4.5
	%	31.0	21.1	70.6	5.6	66.7	34.6	17.3

* Some individuals were in between and were, therefore, classified as half and half.

another preference. Since food itself (amount, kind, wide variety) was the chief reason given for dinner preference, liking food seemed to be associated with meal regularity. Of the three ethnic groups, the Negroes, who showed the greatest tendency to omit meals, also showed less dinner preference.

Both Tables 4-VI and Table 4-VII indicate the high frequency of snacking as a part of the eating pattern of these teenage subjects.

Types of Meals and Snacks

Because types of meals, like meal-eating and snacking patterns, varied considerably, we did not find it possible to choose "typical" meals. The following are illustrations of meals and snacks of subjects who followed the four most common patterns of eating:

1. Three regular, structured meals a day with few snacks:

Caucasian boy aged 16.3 years

Breakfast
   One and one-half cups crushed
      pineapple
   One soft boiled egg
   Two slices toasted cinnamon bread
   One tablespoon butter
   One cup milk
Lunch
   One ham sandwich with mayonnaise and mustard
   One ounce potato chips
   One orange
   Four cookies
   Three cups milk
Dinner (5:30 P.M.)
   Four ounces fried beef liver
   One and one-half cups mashed
      potatoes
   Two tablespoons butter

One-half cup green beans with
   olive oil and lemon juice
Two cups milk
Snack (7:30 P.M.)
   Two and one-half cups ice
      cream

Caucasian girl aged 17.1 years

Breakfast
   One fried egg
   Two slices toast
   One and one-half teaspoons
      butter
   One cup milk
Lunch
   One cheese sandwich
   One apple
Snack (4:20 P.M.)
   Three slices raisin bread
   One tablespoon butter

One apple
One cup skim milk
Dinner
  Two and one-half ounces fried
    fillet of sole
  One-half cup whole kernel corn

One baked potato two inches
  in diameter
One and one-half teaspoons
  butter
One-half cup ice cream
Two cups skim milk

2. Three regular, structured meals a day with many snacks:

Caucasian boy aged 18.1 years

Breakfast (7:00 A.M.)
  One cup dry cereal
  Two tablespoons cream
  One and one-half teaspoons
    sugar
  One doughnut
  One cup low fat milk
Snack (7:50 A.M.)
  Coffee with one teaspoon sugar
Lunch
  Two peanut butter and jelly
    sandwiches
  Six cookies
  One apple
Snack (3:10 P.M.)
  One cup root beer
Dinner (6:45 P.M.)
  One-half cup beef Stroganoff
  One and one-half cups rice
  One cup lettuce salad
Snack (11:00 P.M.)
  One rye wafer
  Two teaspoons butter
  Two apples

Oriental girl aged 15.3 years

Breakfast
  One bologna sandwich with
    mayonnaise and mustard
Lunch
  One bologna sandwich with
    mayonnaise and mustard
  One-third of 29¢ bag potato
    chips
  One can cola drink
Snack (5:00 P.M.)
  One fried egg
  Three slices toast
  One and one-half teaspoons
    butter
  One-half cup milk
Dinner (6:30 P.M.)
  Two cups Spanish rice
Snack (9:00 P.M.)
  Four ounces cola drink
  One piece hard candy
Snack (11:00 P.M.)
  Four ounces cola drink
  Three-fourths cup ice cream

3. One meal a day with additional unstructured meals or snacks:

Negro boy aged 17.1 years

Breakfast—None
Snack (10:40 A.M.)
  One package hard candy
Snack (11:00 A.M.)
  One cup fruit punch

Six peanut butter and cracker
  sandwiches
Snack (1:00 P.M.)
  One candy bar
Snack (2:10 P.M.)
  One candy bar

Dinner (5:45 P.M.)
  Two ounces fried liver
  Two cups bread dressing
  One ear corn on the cob
  One cup lettuce and tomato
    salad with mayonnaise
Snack (9:50 P.M.)
  Six peanut butter and cracker
    sandwiches
Another day from the diary of the
same boy illustrates the contri-
bution of the school lunch:
Breakfast—None
Snack (11:15 A.M.)
  One and one-fourth ounce candy
    covered peanuts
  One and one-fourth ounce salted
    peanuts
  One cup lemonade
Lunch (12:20 P.M.—at school)
  One-eighth of a ten-inch pizza
  One-half cup green beans
  One-half cup carrot and pine-
    apple salad
  One slice French bread with
    butter
  Two tablespoons fruit cocktail
  One cup fruit punch
Snack (12:40 P.M.)
  One cup fruit punch
  One-half apple
Snack (2:15 P.M.)
  One cup fruit punch
Dinner (4:30 P.M.)
  One fried pork chop

One-half cup boiled white beans
One-half cup rice
One and one-half cups milk

Caucasian girl aged 15.8 years
Breakfast—None
Snack (10:30 A.M.)
  Three-fourths cup gelatin des-
    sert
Snack (10:40 A.M.)
  Ten saltine crackers with one
    ounce cheese and one table-
    spoon butter
  Two cups popcorn with two ta-
    blespoons butter
Snack (11:30 A.M.)
  Six ounces skim milk
  One brownie
Snack (2:00 P.M.)
  One-half cup gelatin dessert
  Fifteen green grapes
Snack (2:40 P.M.)
  One ice cream sandwich
Dinner
  Four ounces fried steak
  One-half cup spinach with one
    teaspoon mayonnaise
  Two tablespoons corn
  One-half teaspoon butter
  One-half cup canned peaches
  One ice cream sandwich
Snack (9:20 P.M.)
  Thirteen saltine crackers
  Five ounces chocolate candy
  Six ounces low fat milk

4. Irregular pattern with many snacks and unstructured
meals:

Oriental boy aged 15.8 years

Breakfast
  One-half can turkey-noodle soup
  Tea with four teaspoons sugar
Lunch

Three slices bread
Six teaspoons jam
Snack (4:45 P.M.)
  One slice bread
  Two teaspoons jam
  Two cups sweetened beverage *

* Sweetened beverage refers to a flavoring powder or tablet mixed with water
and sugar.

Snack (6:00 P.M.)
  Four slices bread
  Eight teaspoons jam
  Two apricots
Dinner (7:00 P.M.)
  Seven pieces raw fish (three-
    eighths inch by two inches by
    one inch)
  One cup rice
Snack (11:30 P.M.)
  One hamburger patty

Negro girl aged 16.8 years respon-
sible for her own meal preparation

Breakfast—None
Snack (8:00 A.M.)
  One popsicle

The following, of better nutritional
  quality, is from the diary of a
  Negro boy aged 17.1 years

Breakfast (11:00 A.M.)
  Three fried eggs
  One sausage
  One cup hot chocolate
  Three rolls
  Three tablespoons butter
  One tablespoon jelly
Snack (1:00 P.M.)
  Two cups milk
  One banana
Snack (2:00 P.M.)
  One cup milk
Dinner (5:45 P.M.)
  One hamburger sandwich
  One cup milk
Snack (9:30 P.M.)
  One peanut butter and jelly
    sandwich
  One and one-half cups fruit
    punch
Snack (10:30 P.M.)
  Two cups hot chocolate

Snack (9:34 A.M.)
  One carrot
  One stick celery
Lunch
  One orange
  Two cake doughnuts with choc-
    olate icing
Snack (4:00 P.M.)
  One-half ounce potato chips
  One-half cup corn chips
  One-third cup popcorn
  Three thin pieces salami (four
    and one-half inches diameter)
Dinner (8:40 P.M.)
  One tuna pie
  Twelve ounces cola drink

Many subjects frequently ate meals that did not follow conventional patterns, as illustrated by these meals recorded by different subjects:

Breakfasts

1. Half of one barbecued chicken, potato salad, sweetened beverage,* popsicle
2. Cubed steak, string beans with almond butter, orange juice, scrambled eggs with cheese
3. Pork chop, milk, watermelon, salami, cheese sandwich
4. Boiled potato, hot dog, bread, lemonade, hard cooked egg
5. Fresh peach, applesauce, cheese, toast, raisins, buttermilk

Lunches

1. Milk, cup cakes, popcorn
2. Formula diet drink and chocolate-covered peanuts
3. Potato salad and sunflower seeds
4. Potato chips, candy bar, milk
5. Waffle, cheese, apple, milk

Dinners

1. Pecan pancakes with whipped cream, green salad with ham and cheese, milk
2. Fresh peach, banana, grapenuts with milk, cantaloupe, ice cream, bread with peanut butter
3. Spaghetti with cheese, four scrambled eggs, Canadian bacon, milk, gelatin dessert
4. Hash and sweetened beverage *
5. French fries, catsup, and sweetened beverage *

Snacks were classified in ten categories. The frequency with which these appeared in descending order of popularity were:

Boys	*Girls*
1. Cereal and bread	1. Pie, cake, pastry and cookies
2. Pie, cake, pastry and cookies	2. Candy
3. Soft drinks	3. Fruit
4. Milk	4. Cereals and bread
5. Fruit	5. Soft drinks
6. Eggs, meat, cheese	6. Ice cream
7. Ice cream	7. Milk
8. Candy	8. Eggs, meat, cheese
9. Potato chips	9. Potato chips
10. Vegetables	10. Vegetables

* Sweetened beverage refers to a flavoring powder or tablet mixed with water and sugar.

Vegetable snacks were eaten quite infrequently by all boys and girls. Subjects with differing amounts of body fat did not vary greatly in the types of foods selected for snacks.

Ethnic Origin of Dishes Eaten

Dishes of varying ethnic origin were consumed by subjects of all races, as shown in Table 4-IX. Oriental boys and girls, however, did report a significantly higher number of Oriental dishes than did Negroes and Caucasians. Both Negro and Oriental

TABLE 4–IX

ETHNIC ORIGIN OF FOODS CONSUMED BY RACE—
AVERAGE DISHES PER PERSON FOR FOUR WEEKS

	U. S. South	*Asia*	*Mexico*	*Italy*
		Origin of Dishes		
Boys				
Caucasian	0.3	0.7	2.0	2.4
Negro	1.4	0.2	1.8	2.2
Oriental	0.3	18.8	1.6	3.7
Girls				
Caucasian	0.5	1.6	1.6	2.5
Negro	4.5	2.9	2.7	1.9
Oriental	0.0	27.4	1.4	3.9

youngsters selected foods of Mexican and Italian origin about as frequently as Caucasians did.

Amounts Eaten of Various Food Groups

The average amounts of various food groupings eaten by boys and girls of each body fat class are shown in Table 4-X. Boys ate more of all food groups than girls, and the obese boys and girls ate smaller amounts of dairy products, vegetables, and fruits than other subjects.

Comparisons by race (Table 4-XI) showed that for both sexes Causasians were the greatest consumers of dairy products; fats, oils and nuts; and vegetables and fruits. Negroes led in desserts and sweets. Orientals led in the cereal group and were low in starchy vegetables, since they tended to eat rice rather than potatoes. Of the meat and legume food group, Orientals were the highest consumers among boys, and Negroes among girls.

TABLE 4-X

MEAN GRAMS OF SPECIFIED FOOD GROUPS CONSUMED BY SUBJECTS GROUPED BY SEX AND BODY FAT CLASS
(GRAMS PER DAY FOR FOUR WEEKS)

Food Groups	Boys (N = 61)						Girls (N = 71)					
	All N = 61	Lean N = 9	Somewhat Lean N = 7	Average N = 19	Somewhat Obese N = 9	Obese N = 7	All N = 71	Lean N = 14	Somewhat Lean N = 10	Average N = 31	Somewhat Obese N = 10	Obese N = 6
1. Dairy products	790	729	949	868	678	638	504	593	578	473	478	373
2. Meat, poultry, fish, eggs, and legumes	271	248	302	301	224	249	165	185	182	154	153	168
3. Hydrogenated fats, oils, salad dressings, nuts	24	24	18	24	20	33	19	18	22	20	16	13
4. Cereals, bread, crackers, pastes	254	260	283	270	200	243	152	164	148	156	139	129
5. Vegetables, fruits and juices	481	400	490	561	507	323	408	413	464	394	430	343
6. Desserts and foods primarily sweet *	257	239	245	230	298	315	193	193	194	201	184	171
7. Miscellaneous (soup, gravies, special foods, alcoholic beverages)	98	62	102	131	46	121	53	77	58	44	51	40

* Includes pie, cake, doughnuts, cookies, sweet rolls, candy, syrup, jams, jellies, sugar, soft drinks.

TABLE 4-XI

MEAN GRAMS PER DAY OF SPECIFIED FOOD GROUPS CONSUMED BY SUBJECTS GROUPED BY SEX, ETHNIC ORIGIN, AND SOCIOECONOMIC GROUP

| | Ethnic Origin | | | | | | Socioeconomic Group | | | | | |
| | Boys (N = 51) | | | Girls (N = 71) | | | Boys (N = 51) | | | Girls (N = 71) | | |
Food Groups	Caucasian N = 31	Negro N = 10	Oriental N = 10	Caucasian N = 45	Negro N = 17	Oriental N = 9	Lower Third N = 3	Middle Third N = 27	Upper Third N = 21	Lower Third N = 6	Middle Third N = 39	Upper Third N = 26
1. Dairy products	894	546	800	552	350	550	665	749	859	270	519	534
2. Meat, poultry, fish, eggs, and legumes	273	252	283	158	180	174	230	274	273	173	170	156
3. Hydrogenated fats, oils, salad dressings, nuts	26	23	17	20	14	17	28	22	26	14	21	17
4. Cereals, bread, crackers, pastes	236	214	348	133	163	226	255	252	256	139	167	132
5. Vegetables, fruits and juices	593	301	312	437	342	390	286	402	610	430	404	410
6. Desserts and foods primarily sweet *	265	327	165	181	249	152	257	266	246	218	198	181
7. Miscellaneous (soup, gravies, special foods, alcoholic beverages)	81	45	205	51	39	92	66	121	73	44	56	51

Includes pie, cake doughnuts, cookies, sweet rolls, candy, syrup, jams, jellies, sugar, soft drinks.

Socioeconomic groupings showed that the "upper third" of both sexes used more dairy products. All groups ate generous amounts of the meat and legume group (Table 4-XI). The kinds of meat and other protein-rich foods varied. Oriental boys and girls ate the most fish, while Negroes ate more pork.

The kinds of fruits and vegetables eaten varied by sex, race, and socioeconomic groups. Raw fruits and vegetables were consumed in the greatest quantities by all girls, and cooked fruits and juices were consumed in the largest quantities by the boys. Both were far more popular than either cooked starchy vegetables, or cooked nonstarchy vegetables. The Negro boys and girls and those in the "lower" socioeconomic group ate smaller quantities of raw fruits and vegetables than other boys and girls. Oriental boys and girls ate less of the cooked starchy vegetables and fewer cooked fruits and juices than other boys and girls.

While the boys in the "lower" socioeconomic group ate less of all groups of vegetables and fruits than other boys, the girls in the "lower" socioeconomic group ate less of the raw fruits and vegetables but more cooked starchy and nonstarchy vegetables than other girls. Negro girls were the leading consumers of cooked starchy vegetables, but girls from all ethnic groups consumed about the same amounts of cooked nonstarchy vegetables.

We viewed food groupings also by their caloric contributions. Dairy products and the meat and legume group were the two leading caloric contributors for both sexes and all body fat classes. For the boys, the cereal group was next, followed by desserts and sweets, while the reverse was true for girls.

Most of the fat calories for both boys and girls came from dairy foods (about 30 percent) and meats (30 to 40 percent). Almost twice as many calories came from nuts, oils, and salad dressings as from hydrogenated fats, although these groups contributed a relatively small amount to the total caloric intake.

Both boys and girls got about 15 percent of their carbohydrate from dairy products. Boys got about 30 percent of their carbohydrate from bread, crackers, pasta, cereals and grains and about the same percentage from desserts and foods primarily sweet. Girls got about 26 percent of their carbohydrate from breads, crackers, pasta, cereals, and grains and 34 percent from desserts and foods primarily sweet.

Dairy Products

Generally speaking low calcium intakes accompanied low total caloric intakes, with a smaller number and percentage of calories from the dairy foods. Subjects with low caloric intakes from the dairy group of foods (below 450 calories) tended to have low calcium intakes (below two thirds of the Recommended Dietary Allowances); and subjects with a fairly high caloric intake from the dairy foods (above 700 calories) tended to have high calcium intakes (above Recommended Dietary Allowances). The exceptions to these trends were: those boys and girls who ate large quantities of ice cream and little fluid milk and had low calcium intakes accompanied by a larger caloric contribution from the dairy foods; or those boys and girls who drank skim or low fat milk and ate very little ice cream and so had fairly high calcium intakes with a low intake of calories from the dairy foods.

Among boys and girls with calcium intakes less than two thirds of the Recommended Dietary Allowance, there was a general tendency to substitute soft drinks for milk at meal time.

Coffee

Twenty-five percent of the boys and 39 percent of the girls reported drinking more than one cup of coffee per week. Few, if any, of our subjects could be considered heavy coffee drinkers. The maximum number of cups consumed in any day by any subject was seven; however, this subject drank only 15 cups in four weeks. The subject who drank the most coffee in four weeks consumed an average of two cups per day. In general, coffee did not seem to appear as a substitute for milk for these teenagers.

Vitamin Pills

Nine of the 51 boys and 22 of the 71 girls who kept four weekly food and activity records reported taking vitamin pills one or more times during the four weeks. All were in the "middle" and "upper" socioeconomic classes, and all but one were Caucasian or Oriental. In comparing the group of boys and girls who took vitamin supplements to the entire group, it would appear that their dietary intake of nutrients was similar to the entire sample—or slightly better. As with the entire sample, the most neglected nutrients were calcium and iron, especially for the girls. Since the more common vitamin supplements do not include these minerals, it is doubtful that the supplements increased the adequacy of the nutrient intakes to any degree.

Discussion and Suggestions

Our observation that teenagers tend to omit meals and to snack frequently agrees with the popular impression. Our finding that roughly one third of the subjects and, in particular, 90 percent of the Negro teenagers had highly irregular eating practices during four separate weeks suggests a way of living and eating quite different from the traditional three-meal-a-day pattern. While reasons for this irregularity were not explored in detail, it was apparent that many youngsters were fending for themselves. Some were buying their own snacks while others, as indicated by the "meals" previously described, were apparently helping themselves to whatever they could find in refrigerator or cupboard. Ethnic classification appeared more closely associated than socioeconomic grouping with eating patterns. While there were individual exceptions, those teen-agers who ate regular structured meals, usually augmented by snacks, tended to have better nutrient intakes than these irregular eaters.

Obviously, a change to regular meal eating would necessitate a change in the entire way of life of these children and their families. Is this a realistic and essential goal for nutrition educators? Should home economics and nutritional teaching change its emphasis from meal planning to buying of nutritious snacks and convenience foods? It was apparent that if children were to have nutritious food, it had to be readily available to them.

The gatekeepers to such a food supply were in some instances the children themselves and sometimes the mothers or others in the household. Most in need of help, because of dietary inadequacy, were the obese and the Negro girls.

It is obvious that ethnic food patterns need to be taken into account in nutrition teaching and school lunch programs in the community from which our sample was drawn. It is equally obvious, however, that much intercultural food change has occurred and that stereotyped patterns cannot be assumed.

Nutrient intakes and food patterns both showed that meats and other protein-rich foods were well accepted and consumed in large amounts by those in all ethnic and socioeconomic groups. This group of foods would not seem to require emphasis in nutritional education programs with our population group. Vegetables, on the other hand, were not so regularly consumed.

The failure of vitamin pills to augment low nutrient intakes would seem to show a need for better education regarding their use.

Summary

Results of four seven-day dietary records from a small group of teenagers are reported, as well as seven-day records for a somewhat larger group.

Both from the standpoint of mean nutrient intake levels and percentage of subjects having intakes below two thirds of the Recommended Dietary Allowances, the most neglected nutrients were calcium and iron, particularly for the girls.

The average boys tended to have higher intakes of calories and nutrients than lean or obese boys. The lean girls tended to have a higher intake of calories and nutrients than average or obese girls. In general, a higher caloric intake was associated with a higher intake of protein, minerals, and vitamins.

Negro boys and girls and boys and girls in the lower socioeconomic group tended to have lower intakes of food nutrients than other boys and girls.

There was a tendency for obese boys and girls to eat less frequently than other boys and girls, and also a tendency for the obese or somewhat obese teenagers to skip meals more often than other teenagers. The subjects who ate less than three times a day had poorer diets than others. Those who ate frequently tended to have overall good diets. There was a great range of eating frequency among individual subjects, averaging from two to six times a day over a week's time.

Caloric intake varied greatly from individual to individual, and from day to day for each individual. There was wider variation for each individual from day to day than from week to week.

Boys, but not girls, who were able to mention all of the "Basic Four" food groups tended to have fewer nutrients below the two-thirds Recommended Dietary Allowances level than other boys. There seemed to be no relationship between school performance as measured by grade point averages and quality of the diet as measured by number of nutrients below two-thirds of the Recommended Dietary Allowances.

Four weekly food diaries kept by 122 eleventh and twelfth grade subjects over a period of two years showed marked irregularity in eating practices of approximately one third of the subjects and great variation among subjects, associated to some extent with ethnic and socioeconomic factors.

Snacking was common and tended to benefit nutrient intakes. The meal most frequently skipped was lunch.

Dairy products and the meat and legume group were the two leading calorie contributing groups for both sexes and all body fat classes.

CHAPTER 5

RECORDED ACTIVITIES AND ATTITUDES TOWARD ACTIVITIES*

WHILE ON THE ONE HAND the popular conception of the teenager is that of high levels of physical activity, on the other hand, many technological and cultural changes in the past few decades may have been contributing to a lower level of physical activity for both teenagers and adults. Among these changes are the increased use of the automobile, the popularity and availability of television, and the use of mechanical devices to perform ordinary household and gardening chores.

Our questions then are: How active are teenagers in our eyes? How active are teenagers in their own eyes? Should teenagers be encouraged to be more active? If so, what sorts of activities do they enjoy and approve?

This chapter indicates partial answers to some of these questions.

Other aspects of this study reported in different chapters indicate that teenagers are concerned about obesity, that obesity is already a problem for some, and that the obese teenager does not consume more calories than his nonobese peer. This leads us to the assumption that the obese teenager may have established a pattern of a low level of physical activity that contributes to his obese condition. Can we verify that assumption?

Interviewers checked the food and activity records of the subsample as described in Chapter 2. In checking the records of activity, the interviewers made certain that they understood the

* The substance of this chapter appeared originally in the *Journal of the American Dietetic Association,* 51:433, November 1967. We are indebted to the publication for its use.

TABLE 5–I

CALORIC EXPENDITURE CLASSIFICATION OF
WORK AND EXERCISE

Very Light
(2.5 cal/min; 150 cal/hr)

Standing, at ease	Writing	Light assembly
Lying	Sewing	line
Sitting	Typing	* Talking on phone
Sitting, using arm	Knitting	Playing musical
movements	Light machine	instrument
Reading	work	(* except organ)

Light
(2.5–4.9 cal/min; 150–299 cal/hr)

Personal care	Light gardening	Mixing cement
Walking, slowly	Driving car,	Playing with child
Standing using arm	motorcycle	Pee-wee golfing
movement	Golfing	* Playing organ
Housework, except	Carpentry work	* Driving go-cart
stooping and	Gymnastic exercises,	* Fair rides
bending	except hopping	* Playing baseball
		* Playing ping-pong

Moderate
(5.0–7.4 cal/min; 300–449 cal/hr)

Walking, moderate	Dancing (* Some may be	Pushing wheelbarrow
to fast	Light or Strenuous)	* Washing car
Walking, moderate	Bicycling	* Washing windows
up hill	Bowling	* Roller skating
Housework, stooping	Gymnastic exercises,	* Mowing lawn (not
and bending	hopping and swinging	motorized)
Swimming	arms	* Moving furniture
Heavy gardening	Stacking firewood	* Badminton
Tennis	Using pickaxe	* Lifting weights
		* Pull-ups

Strenuous
(7.5 cal/min; 450 cal/hr)

Running	Digging	Chopping with an
Walking fast up	Sawing wood	axe
hill	Planing wood	Horse riding
Climbing a ladder	Shoveling	* Ice skating
Skiing	Carrying load upstairs	* Basketball (some may
Walking in snow	Playing football	be Light or Moderate

Used by Bureau of Nutrition, California State Department of Public Health, in research on obesity and leanness. (Adapted from R. Passmore and J. Durnin's "Human Energy Expenditure," *Physiological Reviews, 35*:801, 1955).
* Added for School of Public Health research project.
NOTE: Seventy-five steps up are equal to one minute of strenuous activity.

details of each type of activity, i.e. how much time was spent in running, standing, or sitting. The subjects recorded activity by time of day, for example: 7:00 A.M. to 7:15 A.M., ate breakfast; 7:15 to 7:18, brushed teeth; 7:18 to 7:35, read paper. After the interviewer had checked the subject's activity records for detail and accuracy and accounted for any missing time, each time interval was classified as to type of activity performed. The classifications used were sleep, very light (2.5 calories/min), light (2.5 to 4.9 calories/min), moderate (5.0 to 7.4 calories/min) and strenuous (7.5 and more calories/min). These classifications were adapted from the work of Passmore and Durnin (1955) by the Bureau of Nutrition, California State Department of Public Health for their research (Table 5-I) and were kindly shared with us (Hutson *et al.*, 1965). We used them with a few modifications. We asked our subjects to count the number of steps they took going upstairs each day and arbitrarily considered 75 steps up to be the equivalent of one minute of strenuous activity. Although little time might be spent climbing stairs, the contribution of stair-climbing to the day's total energy expenditure might be important.

After the subject's time was classified into various categories to reflect the level of activity participated in during a day, the time for each level of activity was totaled for the week (seven days). A total score was derived by weighing the activity levels in the following manner: time spent in sleep and very light categories was multiplied by a factor of one, light activity by a factor of two, moderate by three, and strenuous by four. This arbitrary scoring was an attempt to give a picture of comparative energy expenditures in a single numerical value.

We classified our subjects by percent of body fat, race, and sex, as described earlier.

Time Spent in Different Activities

Table 5-II shows the time spent in the various classes of activity by boys and girls for all four weeks. During the two summer weeks the subjects were approximately sixteen and seventeen years old. In the spring of 1964 the subjects were approximately 16½ years old and in the spring of 1965 they were about 17½ years.

The significance of differences between arithmetic means was calculated using the standard formulas for large and small sample sizes. In cases where sample size was small and variances differed significantly, a modification of the "t" test was used (1943). A probability level of 0.05 was consistently used.

Sex. The differences between sexes that are statistically

TABLE 5–II

MEANS AND STANDARD DEVIATIONS OF PHYSICAL ACTIVITY
FOR ALL BOYS AND ALL GIRLS FOR FOUR WEEKLY PERIODS

| | Summer, 1963 | | | | Spring, 1964 | | | |
| | Boys (N = 90) | | Girls (N = 94) | | Boys (N = 73) | | Girls (N = 86) | |
	$\bar{X}$	σ	$\bar{X}$	σ	$\bar{X}$	σ	$\bar{X}$	σ
Total Score	222.6	18.59	212.5 †	12.19	211.9	13.65	208.4 †	11.36
Sleep, hrs/wk	65.2 †	7.17	63.5 †	5.77	61.8 †	5.83	61.0 †	8.10
Very light, hrs/wk	64.3 †	12.60	66.2 †	9.09	75.4 †	8.60	75.1 †	8.82
Light, hrs/wk	23.7 *†	8.75	30.4 *†	7.80	20.3 *†	7.43	24.6 *†	6.63
Moderate, hrs/wk	12.0 *	6.88	5.9 *	4.77	7.8 *	4.49	6.1 *	4.49
Strenuous, hrs/wk	2.5 *	2.82	1.1 *	2.09	2.7 *	2.07	1.1 *	1.55

| | Summer, 1964 | | | | Spring, 1965 | | | |
| | Boys (N = 62) | | Girls (N = 82) | | Boys (N = 54) | | Girls (N = 73) | |
	$\bar{X}$	σ	$\bar{X}$	σ	$\bar{X}$	σ	$\bar{X}$	σ
Total Score	215.9	13.48	213.8 †	14.52	216.6	13.69	209.5 †	9.35
Sleep, hrs/wk	64.7 †	7.88	63.8 †	7.52	59.6 †	6.17	58.7 †	5.80
Very light, hrs/wk	67.1 †	14.13	66.6 †	11.11	74.4 †	11.41	76.2 †	7.74
Light, hrs/wk	27.2 †	13.13	30.1 †	8.61	22.1 *†	9.39	25.2 *†	6.84
Moderate, hrs/wk	8.7 *	4.88	6.8 *	5.01	9.1 *	4.40	7.2 *	3.37
Strenuous, hrs/wk	1.2 *	1.61	0.7 *	0.88	2.8 *	2.91	0.7 *	0.84

* Statistically significant differences between sexes for each week.
† Statistically significant differences between 2 spring weeks vs. 2 summer weeks for each sex.

significant show a trend for boys to spend more time in moderate and strenuous activity than girls, and the girls to spend more time in light activity than boys. The total score and time spent by the boys in moderate activity was greater in the summer of 1963 than for any other weekly period. Less time was spent in strenuous activity in the summer of 1964 than in any other week. We might speculate that this was due to increased availability, use of, and interest in the automobile along with the absence of required physical education in the summer.

For the girls the total score was higher in the summer weeks than in the spring weeks, as were the hours spent in sleep.

For both boys and girls the higher very light activity in the spring is probably a reflection of being in school and sitting in class. Also, the greater amount of sleep during the summer weeks is probably due to not having studies to occupy their evenings and being able to sleep later in the mornings.

Particularly striking is the small amount of time spent in moderate and strenuous activity, especially on the part of the girls. In fact, for some of the girls, the only strenuous activity indulged in was stair-climbing.

Body Fat Groups. Table 5-III shows the mean of the four weekly periods of those subjects who completed all four of the

TABLE 5–III

MEAN (FOUR WEEKLY PERIODS) ACTIVITY OF LONGITUDINAL SUBSAMPLE
CLASSIFIED BY BODY FAT

	N		Total Score	Sleep	Very Light	Light	Moderate	Strenuous
					Hours Per Week			
All Boys	51	$\bar{X}$	217.1 *	62.7	70.7	22.9 *	9.5 *	2.5 *
		σ	11.89	5.17	8.69	6.65	3.54	1.52
Lean	9	$\bar{X}$	216.2	62.8	71.6	21.5	9.6	2.4
		σ	10.50	3.94	6.84	6.32	3.36	1.49
Somewhat lean	7	$\bar{X}$	209.3 †	65.7	71.3	22.0	7.7 †	1.3 †
		σ	15.30	5.39	9.24	7.88	4.58	1.17
Average	19	$\bar{X}$	219.2 †	62.4	71.0	22.0	10.4 †	3.0
		σ	10.98	4.43	7.96	5.72	3.15	1.86
Somewhat obese	9	$\bar{X}$	220.7	61.4	68.3	26.5	9.3	2.5 †
		σ	12.22	6.09	13.94	8.91	3.96	0.99
Obese	7	$\bar{X}$	216.2	62.2	70.8	23.4	9.4	2.1
		σ	11.32	7.15	4.74	4.75	3.42	0.69
All Girls	71	$\bar{X}$	210.8 *	61.1	71.7	27.6 *	6.5 *	0.8 *
		σ	8.50	5.02	6.79	5.11	3.18	0.68
Lean	14	$\bar{X}$	209.7	60.3	72.6	28.7	5.4 †‡	0.8
		σ	7.43	4.24	6.11	5.16	1.54	0.47
Somewhat lean	10	$\bar{X}$	212.6	61.9	67.0	27.0	8.1 ‡	0.7 †
		σ	7.67	3.70	4.08	4.52	2.84	0.43
Average	31	$\bar{X}$	210.7	60.2 †	72.9	27.5 †‡	6.3 †	0.9 †
		σ	8.73	4.10	6.16	6.11	3.44	0.73
Somewhat obese	10	$\bar{X}$	209.4	63.5 †	70.8	26.0 ‡	6.6	0.8
		σ	7.24	8.40	11.22	3.29	2.95	0.92
Obese	6	$\bar{X}$	213.6	62.8	68.0	29.2 †	7.1	0.8
		σ	13.68	5.50	5.22	1.84	5.06	0.88

* Statistically significant differences between sexes.
† or ‡ Statistically significant differences between two fat groups so marked within each sex.

weekly diaries (longitudinal subsample) classified by body fat.

Significant differences are those noted in the table and the following: The average boys spend more mean time in strenuous activity than do the somewhat lean, somewhat obese and obese boys; and the larger number of hours spent in light activity by the obese girls than the average, somewhat lean, and somewhat obese girls.

None of these significant differences present any clear-cut indication that the obese teenagers are less active than their nonobese peers, in spite of our findings (Chapter 4) that the obese tend to consume fewer calories than the nonobese. Others (Johnson, Burke and Mayer, 1956; Stefanik, Heald and Mayer, 1959) have found that obese youngsters are less active than the nonobese. As indicated in Chapter 3, the obese boys and girls tended to be the earlier maturers and so perhaps were indeed growing less rapidly. This may have been reflected in their tendency to consume fewer calories. Our obese girls also tended to be the shorter girls throughout their high school years, and so may have needed fewer calories.

Again, the overall inactivity of these teenage subjects is

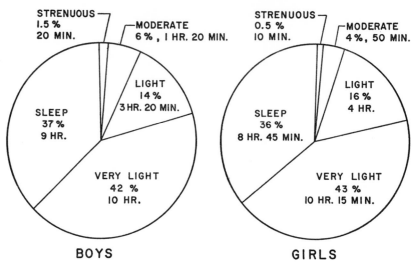

Figure 5–1. Percent and amount of time spent daily in different classes of activity.

clearly shown. For the mean of the four weekly periods, the girls spent more than 95 percent of their time in sleep, very light and light activity, while the boys spent over 90 percent of their time thus (Fig. 5–1). These findings are contrary to the popular idea that the teen years are physically active ones.

RACES. Table 5-IV shows the mean activity of four weekly periods of the longitudinal subsample classified by ethnic origin.

TABLE 5-IV

MEAN (FOUR WEEKLY PERIODS) ACTIVITY OF LONGITUDINAL SUBSAMPLE
CLASSIFIED BY RACE

				Hours Per Week				
Race	*N*		*Total Score*	*Sleep*	*Very Light*	*Light*	*Moderate*	*Strenuous*
Boys								
Caucasian	31	X̄	216.8	62.3	71.4	22.8	9.7	2.3 *
		σ	12.63	5.19	9.31	6.75	3.30	1.39
Negro	10	X̄	220.2	63.5	68.5	22.7	10.0	3.1 *
		σ	14.08	6.15	10.21	7.83	4.78	2.19
Oriental	10	X̄	215.3	63.2	70.6	23.2	8.6	2.3
		σ	6.38	4.41	4.43	5.69	3.05	1.00
Girls								
Caucasian	45	X̄	212.3 *	61.3	71.2 *	27.1 *	7.2 *‡	1.0 *
		σ	9.36	5.22	7.27	5.94	3.41	0.76
Negro	17	X̄	208.9	62.2 *	70.7 †	28.7 *	5.6 *†	0.5 *
		σ	6.70	4.71	5.21	3.25	2.71	0.29
Oriental	9	X̄	207.0 *	58.3 *	76.5 *†	27.7	4.6 †‡	0.7
		σ	4.00	3.80	5.35	3.11	1.22	0.57

* or † or ‡ Significant differences between two races so marked within each sex.

The Negro boys reported a larger number of hours per week in strenuous activity than did the Caucasian boys. Although not statistically significant, there was a tendency for the Negro boys to have higher total scores and higher values for moderate activity than the Caucasian or Oriental boys. This is similar to findings of Hutson and colleagues (1965) about adults in the same geographic area. They found that Negro males were the more physically active group as compared to white males and white females.

The significant differences for the girls indicate a tendency for Caucasian girls to be a more active group than Negro or Oriental girls.

Classification by Caloric Consumption

Since we found that neither low activity levels nor high caloric intakes by themselves corresponded with the obese condition, we wondered if levels of caloric intake might be related to activity levels or other factors involved in the energy balance picture.

We classified our subjects on the basis of various levels of caloric consumption as in Table 5-V. The boys consuming the

TABLE 5–V

VALUES OF SOME PHYSICAL MEASUREMENTS AND ACTIVITY SCORES * CLASSIFIED BY LEVELS OF CALORIC CONSUMPTION * FOR LONGITUDINAL SUBSAMPLE

Calorie Range	N	Mean Height Grade 9 (dm)	Δ † Height (cm)	Δ † LBW (kg)	Δ † TBW (kg)	Total Activity Score
Boys						
1500–2000	4	17.51	2.4	2.92	3.9	217.7
2000–2500	9	16.63	2.5	3.37	3.6	208.3
2500–3000	16	17.20	2.4	3.10	2.7	219.3
3000–3500	11	17.12	3.4	3.45	4.4	221.1
3500–4000	7	17.80	2.5	3.92	5.3	222.4
Girls						
1000–1500	10	16.01	0.1	2.08	3.8	213.6
1500–2000	27	16.26	0.7	0.71	0.6	208.8
2000–2500	27	16.57	0.7	1.03	0.8	211.8
2500–3000	6	16.68	0.5	1.26	2.1	210.6

* Mean values for four weekly periods.
† Mean increase for group from ninth grade to twelfth grade.

most calories did have a higher mean total activity score than the boys consuming fewer calories. We also found that the boys consuming the highest level of calories were taller, gained more in lean body weight and total body weight. The boys consuming the next to the highest level of calories showed the greatest mean gain in height.

The findings for the girls did not agree with those for the boys, in that the girls with the highest activity scores were the ones having the lower level of caloric intake. However, the girls consuming the most calories have the highest mean height, and the girls with the lowest level of caloric consumption have the lowest mean height and the smallest increase in height, but the largest increase in lean body weight and in total body weight.

Self-perception of Activity Level

We have found that these teenagers are not very active by our standards. How active are they according to their own standards?

The foregoing part of this report recorded activity for only a small subsample of our total number of subjects. As previously indicated, our entire sample answered questionnaires each year from the ninth through the twelfth grades. Some of the questions regarded attitudes toward activity.

One of these questions asked students to choose which term of a five-point scale ranging from "very inactive" to "very active" best described them. As shown in Table 5-VI, both sexes at both grade levels checked the "average," "active," and "very active"

TABLE 5-VI

PER CENT OF SUBJECTS CHECKING SPECIFIED RESPONSES TO
QUESTION, "WHICH TERM BEST DESCRIBES YOU?"

	Boys		Girls	
	Ninth Grade (N = 465) %	Twelfth Grade (N = 460) %	Ninth Grade (N = 519) %	Twelfth Grade (N = 379) %
Very inactive	2.8	2.1	1.3	0.2
Inactive	4.1	4.9	4.6	3.3
Average	36.1	29.8	41.6	41.6
Active	35.7	38.0	33.5	35.5
Very active	20.4	22.8	18.7	15.5
No answer	0.9	2.3	0.2	3.8

categories with far greater frequency than the "inactive" and "very inactive." A somewhat greater proportion of boys than girls at both grade levels saw themselves as "very active."

When subjects were divided into body fat classes it was found that proportionately fewer of the "somewhat obese" and "obese" than of the "lean," "somewhat lean," and "average" boys and girls in both the ninth and twelfth grades classified themselves as "active" or "very active," and conversely a greater proportion called themselves "very inactive" and "inactive." These differences, however, were not statistically significant. Girls who considered themselves too fat, although not necessarily found to be so by objective standards, tended to consider themselves above average in activity.

Breakdown by race showed that a smaller percentage of Oriental than of Caucasian or of Negro girls called themselves "active" or "very active," in both the ninth and twelfth grades. Oriental boys, on the other hand, led other races in describing themselves as "active."

Self-perception Compared with Activity Records

We compared the self-perception of our subsample with their activity as reported in their diaries. We found there was a tendency for a larger proportion of our subsample to consider themselves "active" or "very active" than "average." This was also the case for the entire sample. The mean values for total activity scores and time spent in moderate or strenuous activity tended to be larger for those boys and girls who considered themselves above average in activity, as demonstrated by their calling themselves "active" or "very active." Thus, subjects tended to view themselves realistically in relation to their peers.

The majority of subjects considered themselves above average in activity in spite of the fact that the activity level of our subsample was quite low, as measured by the small amount of time spent in either moderate or strenuous activity. This seems to indicate that even though high school students are able to judge their activity level fairly well in relationship to other students, the students' standards for high physical activity levels are rather low.

Perhaps this is a reflection of the low levels of physical

activity of the general population. It also might indicate a tendency on the part of the high school student to confuse being physically active with being "busy"—that is, with having time filled.

Activity Preferences

If we wish to encourage increased physical activity among teenagers in order to form habits that can be carried on into adult life, it is important to know what activities they most enjoy. Also, we were curious to know if there was an association between body composition and the activities preferred.

Students were asked to indicate on a six-point scale patterned after the Louis Guttman (1944) intensity scores how much they liked or disliked each of 28 activities. Lean boys, as a group, had the fewest number of well-liked activities, but the differences between body fat groups were not statistically significant. The activities "liked very much" by the greatest number of students are listed in Table 5-VII. Fewer than half of the activities listed might be classified as requiring only passive participation. As expected, some changes occurred between the ninth and twelfth grades: In the boys' list, dancing and riding in a car replaced watching a ball game and riding a bicycle, while twelfth-grade girls chose reading and boating over cooking and watching TV.

A large proportion of ninth-grade students added a number of their favorites to the 28 activities listed on the questionnaire. Activities mentioned by ninth-grade boys were, in order of decreasing frequency: girls, pool, skating, camping, eating, running, parties, track, hunting, and science. Ninth-grade girls mentioned, in decreasing order: boys, talking on the phone, parties, singing, camping, traveling, skating, drawing and painting, walking, eating, and school. The twelfth-grade questionnaire provided no opportunity for additions.

When ninth-grade favorite activities were grouped according to school attended, we found that swimming, skiing, horseback riding, and boating were mentioned more often by children from the high socioeconomic school than others, possibly because these activities were more readily available.

Although no significant differences were noted in number of

TABLE 5-VII

TEN MOST POPULAR ACTIVITIES OF NINTH- AND TWELFTH-GRADE STUDENTS

	Boys				Girls		
Activity	Ninth Grade (N = 465) %*	Activity	Twelfth Grade (N = 469) %*	Activity	Ninth Grade (N = 519) %*	Activity	Twelfth Grade (N = 394) %*
1. Playing ball	82	1. Sleeping	67	1. Listening to radio or records	81	1. Dancing	75
2. Swimming	71	2. Playing ball	66	2. Dancing	74	2. Listening to radio or records	73
3. Sleeping	63	3. Listening to radio or records	64	3. Swimming	72	3. Watching a movie or play	73
4. Listening to radio or records	63	4. Swimming	52	4. Watching a movie or play	72	4. Sleeping	66
5. Boating	63	5. Watching a movie or play	50	5. Shopping	69	5. Swimming	63
6. Watching TV	59	6. Dancing	50	6. Cooking	65	6. Reading	56
7. Watching a movie or play	57	7. Riding in a car	49	7. Sleeping	62	7. Riding a bicycle	53
8. Watching a ball game	56	8. Boating	48	8. Watching TV	58	8. Boating	53
9. Riding a bicycle	54	9. Playing cards	46	9. Horseback riding	57	9. Shopping	52
10. Playing cards	53	10. Watching TV	44	10. Riding a bicycle	56	10. Horseback riding	52

* Percentage of students who checked "like very much."

well-liked activities of obese and somewhat obese groups and other groups of teenagers, the popularity of certain specific activities differed among the groups of varying body composition. Of the more strenuous physical activities, bowling was checked as "like very much" by more obese than lean boys. The same was true of fishing. Obese girls checked bowling as "like very much" with greater frequency than the lean, while the lean checked skiing more often than obese girls. Playing ball, swimming, and boating were mentioned as well liked by half or more of both obese and lean boys. Over half of the obese and lean girls checked dancing, shopping, swimming, bicycle riding, and playing ball.

At the twelfth-grade level, a greater proportion of obese than lean girls checked ball playing, working, shopping, and fishing as "like very much." More lean than obese checked dancing, boating, and skiing. Swimming was liked by about two thirds of all the girls and bicycle riding, horseback riding, and bowling by about half. Obese boys checked working as very well liked with greater frequency than the lean boys, while the lean outranked them in dancing, boating, skiing, horseback riding, and shopping. Again, swimming was equally popular with both groups, as were ball playing, bicycle riding, bowling and fishing.

It is helpful, in planning programs to encourage increased physical activities, to know that the ten favorite activities of boys and girls at both grade levels include a few that require some physical exertion. Since group activities are not always readily available to out-of-school youth, it is well also that some of these activities can be carried on alone or by a small group.

Summary and Discussion

While gross measurement of physical activity such as we used was probably inadequate to distinguish individual differences in levels of total energy expenditure, it did serve to identify general patterns of activity in the group. Our assessment gave a clear indication that the teenagers studied were fairly inactive.

Our girls averaged more than 95 percent of their time in sleeping, very light, and light activity; our boys averaged more than 90 percent of their time in these categories. Both boys and girls spent on the average nearly 80 percent of their time in combination of sleep and very light activity (less than 2.5 calories per minute). The two most active girls spent approximately 10 percent of their time or about two and one-half hours per day in moderate and strenuous activity. The most active boy spent 13 percent of his time or about three hours per day in moderate and strenuous activity.

This small amount of time may make the relative contribution of moderate and strenuous activities to the total energy expenditure insignificant as compared to differences in basal metabolism and differences in activities requiring very little exertion. Since an average of a little more than ten hours a day was spent in very light activity by both boys and girls, perhaps the differences in the one to one and one-half calories per minute allowable in the categorization of this group of activities could make a great difference in energy expenditure. (The difference of one calorie per minute could amount to 600 calories a day.) Likewise, since our subjects slept on the average of almost nine hours a day and participated in very light activity about ten hours per day, small differences in basal metabolism could amount to large contributions to total energy expenditure.

There are also other factors which may enter into the energy balance picture in addition to caloric consumption and energy expenditure in the form of activity. These might include 1) growth rate, 2) body size which influences basal metabolic rate (BMR) as well as energy expenditure in movement of the total body mass, 3) hormonal and enzymatic differences, 4) hereditary influences and 5) previous history of obesity. In our study, the correlations between caloric intake and height, weight, and lean body weight were all low. This is probably because these factors need to be summed along with those of growth, size, and BMR and weighed differently for different individuals to get any clear picture of energy needs. As indicated in the FAO publication, *Calorie Requirements* (Food and Agriculture Organization of the United States, 1957), it is a fair assumption that 25 percent of the energy expenditure is independent of body weight and 75 percent is directly proportional to body weight either in basal metabolic differences or in energy required to move body mass.

We did find that the groups of boys and girls who consumed the most calories tended to be taller than the other boys and girls. Also, there was a tendency for those boys in the upper ranges of caloric consumption to show larger increases in body height, weight and lean body weight.

Considering both the very large amount of time spent inactively by most subjects and the other factors which may contribute to differences in energy expenditure, it is not too surprising that we found poor correlation between caloric intake and amount of body fat, as well as poor correlation between low level of activity and larger amounts of body fat.

The facts that obesity is a public health problem in the United States and that it occurs in all age groups have been well documented (Metropolitan Life Insurance Co., Nov.–Dec., 1959). The very low level of physical activity observed in this teenage population as well as that seen in an adult population (Hutson *et al.,* 1965) may be a major contributing factor to this obesity. This is further emphasized by our findings, as well as the findings of others, that obese individuals tend to consume fewer, rather than more, calories than do nonobese (Johnson, Burke and Mayer, 1956; Morgan, 1959; Stefanik, Heald and Mayer, 1959).

In comparing our findings on teenagers with those of adults (Hutson *et al.,* 1965), we found that the teenagers spent a little more time in moderate and strenuous activities than did the adults of the same sex. However, the teenagers also spent more of their time in sleeping and very light activity (lying or sitting down) than the adults. It appears that both teenagers and adults are generally sedentary. There are some indications of the preventive aspects of exercise in relationship to cardiovascular disease (Mann *et al.,* 1964). There is also some evidence that a more physically active population is less inclined to become obese (Trulson *et al.,* 1964). And it has been suggested that recommendations for increased physical activity be made to the general population for the purpose of weight control ("The American and his diet," 1964).

These inactive teenagers may be expected to become less physically active as they become adults rather than more so.

In this era of mechanization, few individuals are involved in jobs which require physical exertion. Much more emphasis must be placed on leisure time activities that will contribute to a more physically active way of life. It would appear that habits of active recreational pursuits must be formed and encouraged in the youth of today so that they will want to be more physically active in adulthood.

CHAPTER 6

SCHOOL PERFORMANCE

Physical Performance Scores

THE RELATIONSHIP BETWEEN physical performance and amount of excess body fat was investigated. It was speculated that obese adolescents would do less well in physical performance tests than their peers.

Racial differences in physical performance were investigated as a matter of interest, since all necessary data were available.

Physical performance tests were conducted in the boys' physical education classes of the Berkeley schools during the fall semester, when our subjects were in the ninth, tenth, eleventh, and twelfth grades. Girls were tested only in tenth grade. A description of some of the physical performance tests is given in *The Physical Performance Test for California, 1966* (California State Department of Education, 1966). This same publication gives mean test scores of California students at each grade level (Table 6-I). Certain performance tests done by the Berkeley boys are not included in these statewide norms: running broad jump, football throw, push-up, 440-yard dash, and dips. The sit-up test done by the Berkeley boys differs in

TABLE 6–I

MEAN SCORES MADE BY CALIFORNIA PUPILS IN SPRING 1966
ON PHYSICAL PERFORMANCE TESTS

	AGE (yrs)	Boys								Girls 15	
		14		15		16		17			
		$\bar{X}$	N	$\bar{X}$	N	$\bar{X}$	N	$\bar{X}$	N	$\bar{X}$	N
Standing broad jump (feet)		6.5	448							5.5	336
Pull-ups		6	423	7	342	8	248	9	259		
Sit-ups										30	340
50-yard dash (seconds)		7.0	453							8.0	344
Softball throw (feet)		159	447							84	341
600-yard run-walk (seconds)		135	443							174	320

time limit from that of the 1966 California group; hence scores cannot be compared. Individual test scores were supplied by the physical education teachers.

These data were analysed by computer. The Behrens-Fisher method (Scheffe, 1943) was used when necessitated by small sample size.

NINTH-GRADE BOYS BY BODY FAT CLASSES. Nine physical performance tests were given to ninth-grade boys. The test scores classified by per cent of body fat are given in Table 6-II.

Obese and lean boys had a poorer mean score in the 50-yard dash, running broad jump, and pull-up than the other three fat classes.

In the 600-yard run-walk the somewhat lean boys had a better score than all other fat classes. Obese boys had the poorest mean score.

Obese boys had a poorer score in the standing broad jump and push-up than the other four fat classes.

There were no statistically significant differences between mean scores among fat classes in the softball or football throw, and sit-up test.

The mean scores of the Berkeley boys were equal to or better than the mean scores of the 1966 California group (Table 6-I) in the 50-yard dash, 600-yard run, and standing broad jump. In the pull-up test, the lean and obese scores were much lower than the mean score of the 1966 California norms, but the scores of the other three fat classes were equal to or better than these norms. The softball throw mean scores of the Berkeley boys were slightly lower than the 1966 California norms.

NINTH-GRADE BOYS BY RACE. In Table 6-III, performance test data for ninth-grade boys classified by race are presented.

In the 50-yard dash Negro boys had the best score, Oriental boys the next best, and Caucasians the poorest.

Oriental boys had the best scores in the 600-yard run-walk; the difference between Caucasian and Negro scores was statistically insignificant.

Standing broad jump scores showed no racial differences.

Negro boys had a better score in the running broad jump than the Caucasians and Orientals.

TABLE 6-II

PHYSICAL PERFORMANCE SCORES OF NINTH-GRADE BOYS CLASSIFIED BY BODY FAT CLASSES

Fat Classes	50-Yard Dash (Seconds)			600-Yard Run-Walk (Seconds)			Standing Broad Jump (Feet)		
	X	σ	N	X	σ	N	X	σ	N
Lean	7.2	0.43	30	118.7	12.49	28	6.5	0.56	21
Somewhat lean	7.0	0.50	49	111.5	10.72	50	6.6	0.67	41
Average	7.0	0.57	164	115.7	19.23	161	6.7	0.87	136
Somewhat obese	7.0	0.62	51	120.1	14.29	50	6.6	0.95	44
Obese	7.2	0.56	32	131.8	25.65	29	6.2	0.55	24

Fat Classes	Running Broad Jump (Feet)			Football Throw (Feet)			Softball Throw (Feet)		
	X	σ	N	X	σ	N	X	σ	N
Lean	12.2	1.54	25	86.3	23.47	28	154.7	34.58	28
Somewhat lean	13.3	1.67	34	86.3	20.05	45	152.9	27.95	45
Average	13.0	1.90	99	90.1	21.68	151	160.2	35.49	148
Somewhat obese	13.1	1.71	28	89.6	25.54	44	155.8	35.68	45
Obese	11.6	2.22	16	90.3	29.92	29	158.0	34.50	21

Fat Classes	Push-ups (Number)			Pull-ups (Number)			Sit-ups (Number)		
	X	σ	N	X	σ	N	X	σ	N
Lean	24.7	11.94	28	3.5	2.50	24	22.6	3.62	29
Somewhat lean	29.5	12.19	48	6.2	3.74	38	22.8	2.90	49
Average	28.7	14.17	151	6.2	3.89	135	23.3	3.28	162
Somewhat obese	24.9	14.15	43	7.0	4.69	35	23.1	3.70	51
Obese	17.8	8.74	24	3.6	1.35	15	21.9	3.26	31

TABLE 6-III

PHYSICAL PERFORMANCE SCORES OF NINTH-GRADE BOYS CLASSIFIED BY RACE

RACE	50-Yard Dash (Seconds)			600-Yard Run-Walk (Seconds)			Standing Broad Jump (Feet)		
	X	σ	N	X	σ	N	X	σ	N
Caucasian	7.2	0.58	202	119.0	20.66	197	6.6	0.89	183
Negro	6.8	0.49	105	115.1	15.33	101	6.5	0.77	66
Oriental	6.9	0.31	31	115.0	6.33	31	6.8	0.54	29

RACE	Running Broad Jump (Feet)			Football Throw (Feet)			Softball Throw (Feet)		
	X	σ	N	X	σ	N	X	σ	N
Caucasian	12.6	1.83	141	84.2	23.06	185	153.4	36.03	171
Negro	13.4	1.96	65	98.4	22.54	94	165.0	31.91	98
Oriental	12.5	0.99	12	83.1	17.13	30	152.3	24.60	27

RACE	Push-ups (Number)			Pull-ups (Number)			Sit-ups (Number)		
	X	σ	N	X	σ	N	X	σ	N
Caucasian	27.6	13.90	187	5.7	3.88	148	22.3	3.09	205
Negro	23.6	11.18	92	6.4	3.85	84	24.2	3.46	102
Oriental	33.0	13.94	29	5.1	3.49	24	23.1	2.69	31

In both the football and softball throw, Negro boys had a better score than the other two racial groups.

Oriental boys had the highest score in the push-up test, Caucasians the next highest, and Negroes the lowest.

Pull-up scores showed no statistically significant racial differences.

Negro boys had a better sit-up score than Caucasian boys, while the Orientals' score did not differ significantly from either of the other racial groups.

Mean scores of the Berkeley boys in the 50-yard dash, the 600-yard run-walk, softball throw, standing broad jump, and pull-ups were approximately the same as the mean scores of the 1966 California group (California State Department of Education, 1966).

TENTH-GRADE GIRLS BY BODY FAT CLASSES. Physical performance scores of tenth-grade girls classified by percent of body fat are given in Table 6-IV.

The mean scores of the obese girls in the 50-yard dash, 600-yard run-walk, and standing broad jump were poorer than all other fat classes, and statistically different from the somewhat lean, average, and somewhat obese classes.

The softball throw scores did not follow this trend. The score of the obese girls was poor, but not as poor as that of the lean class. The lean girls had a mean score that was statistically poorer than that of the average and somewhat obese girls.

When the mean scores of the Berkeley girls were compared with the 1966 California group mean scores, the obese girls had poorer scores in all the performance tests.

In the 50-yard dash and the standing broad jump the mean scores of all fat classes except the obese were approximately equal to the mean scores of the 1966 California group. Mean score in the 600-yard run-walk of the somewhat lean girls was better than the mean score of the 1966 California group; the score of the average girls was approximately equal; the other three fat classes had poorer scores. Mean softball throw scores of the average and somewhat obese girls were equal to the California norms. The scores of the other fat classes were poorer. All fat classes except the obese had higher mean numbers of

TABLE 6-IV

PHYSICAL PERFORMANCE SCORES OF TENTH-GRADE GIRLS

CLASSIFIED BY BODY FAT CLASSES

Fat Classes	50-Yard Dash (Seconds)			600-Yard Run-Walk (Seconds)			Standing Broad Jump (Feet)			Softball Throw (Feet)			Sit-ups (Number)		
	X̄	σ	N	X̄	σ	N	X̄	σ	N	X̄	σ	N	X̄	σ	N
Lean	8.1	0.84	28	171.3	27.31	26	5.4	0.48	28	71.6	22.05	22	30.3	10.42	27
Somewhat lean	7.8	0.65	44	160.9	26.94	38	5.3	0.76	45	78.6	26.64	39	31.2	9.68	45
Average	7.9	0.69	146	169.1	37.72	134	5.5	0.72	155	83.4	24.81	119	32.5	10.03	157
Somewhat obese	8.0	0.62	42	173.0	25.80	39	5.2	0.67	41	84.7	23.28	36	34.0	12.08	43
Obese	8.3	0.74	26	215.6	64.23	23	4.9	0.73	28	75.6	24.19	15	25.1	14.41	28

CLASSIFIED BY RACE

Race	50-Yard Dash (Seconds)			600-Yard Run-Walk (Seconds)			Standing Broad Jump (Feet)			Softball Throw (Feet)			Sit-ups (Number)		
	X̄	σ	N	X̄	σ	N	X̄	σ	N	X̄	σ	N	X̄	σ	N
Caucasian	8.0	0.69	187	167.5	31.03	173	5.3	0.74	195	77.4	22.85	162	33.0	11.19	195
Negro	7.7	0.68	79	189.0	61.25	68	5.5	0.72	82	96.6	24.77	55	30.6	11.32	85
Oriental	8.2	0.60	25	177.8	25.21	24	5.3	0.49	26	73.9	16.49	18	26.8	10.66	26

sit-ups than the 1966 California group. The obese followed their overall trend of poorer scores.

TENTH-GRADE GIRLS BY RACE. In Table 6-IV, physical performance scores of tenth-grade girls have been classified by race.

Negro girls had a statistically better score than the Caucasians and Orientals in the 50-yard dash, standing broad jump, and softball throw.

Caucasian girls had a better score in the 600-yard run-walk than Negro girls, while the Orientals' score did not differ significantly from either of the other races.

The sit-up score of the Caucasian girls was statistically better than that of the Orientals, while the Negro score was between the other scores and did not differ statistically from either.

The Negro girls had mean scores that were equal to or better than the scores of the 1966 California group (Table 6-I) in the 50-yard dash, standing broad jump, and the softball throw. The scores of the other races were poorer than the California norms in these events. The 600-yard run-walk score of the Caucasians was equal to the score of the 1966 California group, while the other races had poorer scores.

The mean sit-up score of the Caucasian girls was higher than the California norm; that of the Negro girls was approximately equal to it; the Orientals' score was poorer.

TENTH-GRADE BOYS BY BODY FAT CLASSES. Table 6-V gives physical performance scores classified by percent of body fat for the four tests administered to tenth-grade boys.

In the 440-yard dash the obese boys had the poorest score of the five fat classes. Their score was statistically lower than the score of the average boys; no other differences among fat classes were statistically significant.

In the pull-up test the obese and somewhat obese boys had poorer mean scores than the other three fat classes. The scores of the lean and average boys were statistically higher than the score of the somewhat obese boys.

There were no significant differences among the fat classes in mean number of sit-ups performed. The obese did as well as the other classes in this test.

In the push-up test the score of the obese group was statistically poorer than all other fat classes.

TABLE 6-V

PHYSICAL PERFORMANCE SCORES OF TENTH-GRADE BOYS

CLASSIFIED BY BODY FAT CLASSES

Fat Classes	440-Yard Dash (Seconds)			Pull-ups (Number)			Sit-ups (Number)			Push-ups (Number)		
	X̄	σ	N	X̄	σ	N	X̄	σ	N	X̄	σ	N
Lean	73.9	7.13	10	10.7	6.10	11	42.2	3.19	12	28.9	11.52	13
Somewhat lean	70.8	5.44	13	8.9	4.07	14	40.2	5.15	16	29.6	10.73	15
Average	73.5	8.42	53	10.0	6.26	58	41.1	6.13	57	27.0	10.58	68
Somewhat obese	76.0	9.54	14	6.6	5.72	15	40.9	5.35	16	25.0	10.22	18
Obese	89.5	16.08	17	6.9	6.84	13	39.4	6.64	19	19.3	9.09	18

CLASSIFIED BY RACE

Race	440-Yard Dash (Seconds)			Pull-ups (Number)			Sit-ups (Number)			Push-ups (Number)		
	X̄	σ	N	X̄	σ	N	X̄	σ	N	X̄	σ	N
Caucasian	76.0	11.09	47	8.7	7.28	48	39.1	6.21	55	25.4	11.93	60
Negro	74.3	11.02	46	10.0	5.05	51	42.7	4.91	52	25.9	8.93	56
Oriental	79.4	7.40	12	6.5	4.23	11	40.2	4.60	13	30.8	10.26	14

In the pull-up test all fat classes of Berkeley boys did as well or better than the mean California norm.

TENTH-GRADE BOYS BY RACE. A racial breakdown of the tenth-grade boys' performance scores is given in Table 6-V.

There were no trends or significant differences among the races in the 440-yard dash.

In the pull-up test the score of the Negro boys was higher than the score of the Caucasians, which in turn was higher than that of the Oriental boys. The Oriental score was significantly lower than that of the other two races.

Again in the sit-up test the Negro boys had the highest score. Their score was statistically higher than that of the Caucasians, but not of the Orientals.

Oriental boys had the highest score in the push-up test. Their score was statistically higher than that of the Negroes.

The Berkeley Negro boys had a mean pull-up score that was higher than that of the 1966 California group, as did the Caucasians. The Oriental score was slightly below the California norm.

ELEVENTH-GRADE BOYS BY BODY FAT CLASSES. Physical performance scores of eleventh-grade boys classified by percent of body fat are given in Table 6-VI.

In the 440-yard dash, pull-up, and dip tests the obese boys had statistically poorer scores than did all other fat classes. There were no statistically significant differences among the scores of the four other fat classes.

The obese boys had the poorest score in the sit-up test also. Their score was statistically lower than that of the somewhat lean, average, and somewhat obese classes.

All fat classes except the obese had better mean scores in the pull-up test than did the 1966 California group.

ELEVENTH-GRADE BOYS BY RACE. Table 6-VI gives the physical performance scores of eleventh-grade boys classified by race.

The 440-yard dash and sit-up scores did not reveal any racial differences.

Negro boys had the best pull-up score, which was statistically higher than that of the Orientals.

In the dip test the scores of the three races did not differ

TABLE 6-VI

PHYSICAL PERFORMANCE SCORES OF ELEVENTH-GRADE BOYS

CLASSIFIED BY BODY FAT CLASSES

Fat Classes	440-Yard Dash (Seconds)			Pull-ups (Number)			Sit-ups (Number)			Dips (Number)		
	X̄	σ	N	X̄	σ	N	X̄	σ	N	X̄	σ	N
Lean	72.5	7.88	30	9.5	4.17	30	45.1	5.60	33	11.7	5.50	31
Somewhat lean	69.4	9.45	46	10.0	3.77	51	46.7	8.70	50	12.2	4.90	49
Average	69.0	5.97	161	10.6	4.54	170	46.7	5.73	173	12.3	6.45	169
Somewhat obese	71.6	8.82	46	9.9	4.95	46	46.1	5.62	47	12.1	6.58	45
Obese	77.9	9.22	26	7.0	4.54	29	42.6	6.79	35	8.8	5.16	30

CLASSIFIED BY RACE

Race	440-Yard Dash (Seconds)			Pull-ups (Number)			Sit-ups (Number)			Dips (Number)		
	X̄	σ	N	X̄	σ	N	X̄	σ	N	X̄	σ	N
Caucasian	70.5	8.03	178	9.8	4.63	183	46.2	6.72	192	11.7	5.93	184
Negro	69.8	6.74	89	10.6	4.21	97	46.1	6.04	96	11.9	6.19	98
Oriental	72.7	9.82	27	9.2	4.64	32	46.6	5.98	33	13.2	6.75	30

TABLE 6-VII

PHYSICAL PERFORMANCE SCORES OF TWELFTH-GRADE BOYS

CLASSIFIED BY BODY FAT CLASSES

Fat Classes	440-Yard Dash (Seconds)			Pull-ups (Number)			Sit-ups (Number)			Dips (Number)		
	X	σ	N	X	σ	N	X	σ	N	X	σ	N
Lean	70.0	8.33	35	10.8	4.22	32	40.7	12.32	34	19.1	13.84	33
Somewhat lean	68.6	5.87	50	10.4	4.26	52	44.8	8.87	46	16.1	9.16	47
Average	68.5	7.13	152	11.4	4.82	161	44.4	11.66	146	18.9	11.76	154
Somewhat obese	70.7	9.59	44	10.6	5.30	45	44.4	9.56	47	18.3	10.06	47
Obese	76.0	6.59	25	5.6	4.66	24	44.6	9.69	31	12.0	9.37	30

CLASSIFIED BY RACE

Race	440-Yard Dash (Seconds)			Pull-ups (Number)			Sit-ups (Number)			Dips (Number)		
	X	σ	N	X	σ	N	X	σ	N	X	σ	N
Caucasian	69.7	7.29	223	10.0	5.31	220	43.4	11.30	210	17.0	11.63	207
Negro	68.1	7.13	109	12.0	4.61	120	43.1	12.34	121	20.3	12.17	129
Oriental	71.5	13.58	40	10.2	4.65	40	46.5	6.57	37	16.9	8.42	38

statistically; however, the Oriental mean was somewhat higher than those of the other two races.

The Berkeley boys had higher mean pull-up scores than did the 1966 California group.

TWELFTH-GRADE BOYS BY BODY FAT CLASSES. Table 6-VII gives physical performance scores of twelfth-grade boys classified by percent of body fat.

The 440-yard dash score of the obese group was statistically poorer than the scores of lean, somewhat lean, and average boys.

Obese boys had statistically poorer scores than all other fat classes in the pull-up and dip tests.

In the sit-up test, however, there were no significant differences in mean scores among the fat classes. The obese group performed just as well as the other fat classes.

When the pull-up scores of the Berkeley group were compared with the 1966 California group, all fat classes except the obese had slightly higher mean scores than the California norms. The obese score was considerably lower than the 1966 norms.

TWELFTH-GRADE BOYS BY RACE. Physical performance scores of twelfth-grade Berkeley boys classified by race are given in Table 6-VII.

No significant racial differences appeared in the 440-yard dash.

The pull-up and dip scores of the Negro boys were statistically better than those of the other two races.

Oriental boys had a statistically better score than Caucasian and Negro boys in the sit-up test.

The three Berkeley racial groups had better mean pull-up scores than the 1966 California group.

Effect of Increase in Age on Physical Performance Scores of Boys

The pull-up test was the only test which was given to the boys for the four consecutive years for which we collected data. Scores were available for the sit-up and 440-yard dash tests in tenth, eleventh, and twelfth grades for boys. These data are given in Tables 6-VIII, 6-IX, and 6-X.

BODY FAT CLASSES. Pull-ups: There was a significant improve-

TABLE 6-VIII

PULL-UP SCORES OF NINTH-, TENTH-, ELEVENTH-, AND TWELFTH-GRADE BOYS CLASSIFIED BY BODY FAT CLASSES AND RACE

	Ninth Grade			Tenth Grade			Eleventh Grade			Twelfth Grade		
	$\bar{X}$	σ	N	$\bar{X}$	σ	N	$\bar{X}$	σ	N	$\bar{X}$	σ	N
Fat Classes												
Lean	3.5	2.50	24	10.7	6.10	11	9.5	4.17	30	10.8	4.22	32
Somewhat lean	6.2	3.74	38	8.9	4.07	14	10.0	3.77	51	10.4	4.26	52
Average	6.2	3.89	135	10.0	6.26	58	10.6	4.54	170	11.4	4.82	161
Somewhat obese	7.0	4.69	35	6.6	5.72	15	9.9	4.95	46	10.6	5.30	45
Obese	3.6	1.35	15	6.9	6.84	13	7.0	4.54	29	5.6	4.66	24
Race												
Caucasian	5.7	3.88	148	8.7	7.28	48	9.8	4.63	183	10.0	5.31	220
Negro	6.4	3.85	84	10.0	5.05	51	10.6	4.21	97	12.0	4.61	120
Oriental	5.1	3.49	24	6.5	4.23	11	9.2	4.64	32	10.2	4.65	40

TABLE 6–IX

PHYSICAL PERFORMANCE SCORES CLASSIFIED BY BODY FAT
CLASSES OF TENTH-, ELEVENTH-, AND TWELFTH-GRADE BOYS

	Tenth Grade			Eleventh Grade			Twelfth Grade		
Fat Classes	$\bar{X}$	σ	N	$\bar{X}$	σ	N	$\bar{X}$	σ	N
Sit-ups (number)									
Lean	42.2	3.19	12	45.1	5.60	33	40.7	12.32	34
Somewhat lean	40.2	5.15	16	46.7	8.70	50	44.8	8.87	46
Average	41.1	6.13	57	46.7	5.73	173	44.4	11.66	146
Somewhat obese	40.9	5.35	16	46.1	5.62	47	44.4	9.56	47
Obese	39.4	6.64	19	42.6	6.79	35	44.6	9.69	31
440-Yard Dash (seconds)									
Lean	73.9	7.13	10	72.5	7.88	30	70.0	8.33	35
Somewhat lean	70.8	5.44	13	69.4	9.45	46	68.6	5.87	50
Average	73.5	8.42	53	69.0	5.97	161	68.5	7.13	152
Somewhat obese	76.0	9.54	14	71.6	8.82	46	70.7	9.59	44
Obese	89.5	16.08	17	77.9	9.22	26	76.0	6.59	25

ment in test scores between ninth and tenth grades, after which
the scores remained approximately the same for all fat classes
except the somewhat obese. The improvement in this class took
place between the tenth and eleventh grades. The obese group
followed the general trend, with the exception of the twelfth-
grade mean score, which declined from the eleventh-grade mean
(Table 6-VIII).

Sit-ups: There was a slight improvement in mean scores for
all fat classes between tenth and eleventh grades; changes be-

TABLE 6–X

PHYSICAL PERFORMANCE SCORES CLASSIFIED BY RACE OF
TENTH-, ELEVENTH- AND TWELFTH-GRADE BOYS

	Tenth Grade			Eleventh Grade			Twelfth Grade		
Race	$\bar{X}$	σ	N	$\bar{X}$	σ	N	$\bar{X}$	σ	N
Sit-ups (number)									
Caucasian	39.1	6.21	55	46.2	6.72	192	43.4	11.30	210
Negro	42.7	4.91	52	46.1	6.04	96	43.1	12.34	121
Oriental	40.0	4.60	13	46.6	5.98	33	46.5	6.57	37
440-Yard Dash (seconds)									
Caucasian	76.0	11.09	47	70.5	8.03	178	69.7	7.29	223
Negro	74.3	11.02	46	69.7	6.74	89	68.1	7.13	109
Oriental	79.4	7.40	12	72.7	9.82	27	71.5	13.58	40

tween eleventh and twelfth grades were insignificant (Table 6-IX).

440-yard dash: Mean scores improved slightly each year for all fat classes. The improvement was most pronounced for the obese group between tenth and eleventh grades (Table 6-IX).

RACE. Pull-ups: Scores of the Caucasian boys improved significantly between ninth and tenth grades, but not thereafter. The mean scores of the Negro boys improved significantly between ninth and tenth grades and between eleventh and twelfth grades. The mean scores of the Orientals improved slightly each year; the biggest improvement was between tenth and eleventh grades (Table 6-X).

Sit-ups: The mean scores of all races improved between tenth and eleventh grades, but dropped significantly for the Caucasian and Negro boys between eleventh and twelfth grades. There was no change in mean scores for the Orientals between eleventh and twelfth grades (Table 6-X).

440-yard dash: All races improved their mean test scores significantly between tenth and eleventh grades, but there was no improvement between eleventh and twelfth grades for any race (Table 6-X).

Performance and Obesity

The obese boys tended to do less well in the physical performance tests than the other boys. The sit-up test was the only exception; in this, they did as well as the other fat classes in all grades except eleventh. In ninth grade they equalled the mean score of other fat classes in both the softball and football throw tests.

There was a tendency in the ninth grade for the lean boys to do poorly in the performance tests also. This tendency disappeared in the higher grades.

Obese girls followed the trend of the obese boys in their performance scores; they did less well than other fat classes.

There were no clear-cut racial trends in the physical performance test scores for either sex. Often the Negro boys had the best mean score, but only in the pull-up test did the Negroes consistently have the best scores.

Grades and Absences

The relationship between amount of excess body fat and academic performance as measured by the semester grade averages of our students was investigated, as were physical education grades.

The relationship between the number of days of excused and unexcused absences and body fat, race, and socioeconomic level were studied also. Unexcused absences were known to be not due to illness; excused absences, on the other hand, were likely to have been due to illness but not necessarily so. Several studies (Hinkle *et al.*, 1957; Murphy *et al.*, 1962) have noted that persons with emotional and social problems have a high incidence of minor illnesses.

Semester grade averages, physical education grades, and number of days of excused and unexcused absences were supplied by the Berkeley Unified School District for the fall semesters of the 1962, 1963, and 1964 school years, when the students were in the tenth, eleventh, and twelfth grades, respectively. Such data were not obtained for the ninth grade.

The grading system used in the Berkeley schools is: A = 4.0, B = 3.0, C = 2.0, D = 1.0, F = 0.0.

The data for each semester were separated by sex, and then by body fat class, racial group, and socioeconomic level by census tract as described in Chapter 2.

Semester Grade Averages

Semester grade averages for tenth, eleventh, and twelfth grades classified by percent of body fat are shown in Table 6-XI. Semester grade averages tended to be lower for obese boys, but differences were not statistically significant. For girls, however, the semester grade averages of the obese were statistically lower than all other fat classes for all three years.

Racial classification of semester grade averages (Table 6-XII) revealed definite trends. Orientals had the highest mean averages, Caucasians the next highest, and Negroes the lowest. This pattern applied to both boys and girls for all three grades; all differences are statistically significant (0.05 level).

TABLE 6–XI

SEMESTER GRADE AVERAGES CLASSIFIED BY
PERCENT OF BODY FAT

FAT CLASSES	Tenth Grade			Eleventh Grade			Twelfth Grade		
	$\bar{X}$	σ	N	$\bar{X}$	σ	N	$\bar{X}$	σ	N
	Boys								
Lean	2.10	0.784	43	2.29	0.686	38	2.46	0.642	38
Somewhat lean	2.36	0.803	63	2.19	0.773	55	2.48	0.749	56
Average	2.23	0.778	214	2.22	0.738	188	2.37	0.758	189
Somewhat obese	2.10	0.813	68	2.02	0.768	55	2.31	0.788	60
Obese	1.90	0.659	41	2.03	0.726	39	2.14	0.837	36
	Girls								
Lean	2.67	0.667	42	2.43	0.674	36	2.77	0.712	39
Somewhat lean	2.48	0.791	65	2.56	0.738	54	2.74	0.640	59
Average	2.40	0.773	210	2.37	0.753	170	2.70	0.708	191
Somewhat obese	2.16	0.630	67	2.34	0.699	54	2.68	0.712	59
Obese	1.80	0.687	43	2.09	0.635	33	2.17	0.712	35

TABLE 6–XII

SEMESTER GRADE AVERAGES CLASSIFIED BY RACE

RACE	Tenth Grade			Eleventh Grade			Twelfth Grade		
	$\bar{X}$	σ	N	$\bar{X}$	σ	N	$\bar{X}$	σ	N
	Boys								
Caucasian	2.42	0.773	255	2.34	0.816	254	2.55	0.744	250
Negro	1.67	0.661	163	1.66	0.588	154	1.96	0.708	155
Oriental	2.45	0.645	40	2.54	0.587	39	2.62	0.638	39
	Girls								
Caucasian	2.55	0.740	267	2.53	0.752	250	2.86	0.622	238
Negro	1.81	0.568	152	1.90	0.663	144	2.12	0.752	124
Oriental	2.74	0.552	37	2.60	0.524	37	3.01	0.476	35

Classification of semester grade averages (Table 6-XIII) by socioeconomic level shows that for both sexes in each grade those in the upper-third level had semester averages that were statistically higher than those of the other two levels. The middle-third level had statistically higher semester averages than the lower-third level for both sexes at each grade except twelfth-grade boys.

Physical Education Grades

Physical education grades for tenth, eleventh, and twelfth grades classified by percent of body fat (Table 6-XIV) indi-

TABLE 6–XIII

SEMESTER GRADE AVERAGES CLASSIFIED BY
SOCIOECONOMIC LEVEL

SOCIO-ECONOMIC LEVEL	Tenth Grade			Eleventh Grade			Twelfth Grade		
	X̄	σ	N	X̄	σ	N	X̄	σ	N
	Boys								
Lower-third	1.83	0.586	67	1.86	0.645	49	2.34	1.250	62
Middle-third	2.22	0.671	175	2.08	0.735	204	2.30	1.016	238
Upper-third	2.76	0.620	144	2.47	0.670	122	2.55	0.828	161
	Girls								
Lower-third	1.86	0.635	36	1.85	0.619	35	2.22	0.862	48
Middle-third	2.27	0.700	196	2.36	0.696	192	2.66	0.890	211
Upper-third	2.77	0.642	120	2.55	0.739	120	2.90	0.850	139

TABLE 6–XIV

PHYSICAL EDUCATION SEMESTER GRADES CLASSIFIED
BY PERCENT BODY FAT

FAT CLASSES	Tenth Grade			Eleventh Grade			Twelfth Grade		
	X̄	σ	N	X̄	σ	N	X̄	σ	N
	Boys								
Lean	2.59	0.964	42	2.61	1.326	38	2.03	1.241	38
Somewhat lean	2.93	1.013	63	2.33	1.262	55	2.30	1.159	56
Average	2.83	1.114	215	2.49	1.230	188	2.43	1.298	190
Somewhat obese	2.59	1.095	66	2.16	1.411	55	2.16	1.267	61
Obese	1.95	1.080	42	1.87	1.217	39	1.86	1.058	37
	Girls								
Lean	2.97	0.935	41	2.77	1.031	35	2.82	0.885	39
Somewhat lean	2.93	1.013	65	2.74	1.131	54	2.78	0.872	59
Average	2.69	1.033	209	2.41	1.082	167	2.73	0.946	193
Somewhat obese	2.70	0.953	67	2.33	1.133	54	2.78	0.892	59
Obese	2.02	1.219	42	2.15	1.064	33	2.20	0.833	35

cated that obese boys tend to have lower grades than do boys in other fat classes. Grades' of the girls followed the same pattern.

When physical education grades were classified by race (Table 6–XV), statistical analyses showed that for both sexes Caucasians and Orientals had higher grades than Negroes in tenth grade, while in eleventh and twelfth grades Orientals had the highest physical education grades, Caucasians the next highest, and Negroes the lowest mean grade.

TABLE 6–XV

PHYSICAL EDUCATION SEMESTER GRADES
CLASSIFIED BY RACE

RACE	Tenth Grade			Eleventh Grade			Twelfth Grade		
	$\bar{X}$	σ	N	$\bar{X}$	σ	N	$\bar{X}$	σ	N
	Boys								
Caucasian	2.96	1.019	256	2.55	1.246	254	2.42	1.232	251
Negro	2.12	1.111	162	1.58	1.302	154	1.80	1.286	155
Oriental	3.15	0.879	39	3.05	0.724	39	2.77	1.038	39
	Girls								
Caucasian	2.97	0.945	266	2.58	1.016	245	2.84	0.934	240
Negro	1.98	0.976	149	1.74	1.147	144	2.32	0.907	124
Oriental	3.14	0.822	37	3.08	0.640	37	2.89	0.900	35

Grouping physical education grades by socioeconomic levels (Table 6-XVI) resulted in a definite trend toward lower grades for the lower socioeconomic level for both sexes. Other statistically significant differences follow. The male upper-third level had the highest mean grade all three years, and in tenth and eleventh grades the middle third's mean grade fell between the other levels. For the girls, only in the tenth grade did the mean physical education grades differ significantly from one another. In eleventh and twelfth grades the upper- and middle-third level grades did not differ significantly; however, both were higher than the lower-third level.

TABLE 6–XVI

PHYSICAL EDUCATION SEMESTER GRADES CLASSIFIED
BY SOCIOECONOMIC LEVEL

SOCIO-ECONOMIC LEVEL	Tenth Grade			Eleventh Grade			Twelfth Grade		
	$\bar{X}$	σ	N	$\bar{X}$	σ	N	$\bar{X}$	σ	N
	Boys								
Lower-third	2.29	1.004	66	1.67	1.329	49	1.98	1.204	62
Middle-third	2.83	0.970	174	2.23	1.260	204	2.14	1.311	238
Upper-third	3.33	0.712	144	2.88	1.110	122	2.48	1.230	161
	Girls								
Lower-third	2.03	1.108	36	1.77	1.215	35	2.35	0.838	48
Middle-third	2.59	1.021	194	2.47	1.062	190	2.68	0.955	211
Upper-third	3.18	0.816	120	2.65	1.007	118	2.86	0.870	139

School Attendance Records

BODY FAT CLASSES. School attendance records classified by percent of body fat are shown in Table 6-XVII.

Differences between fat classes in percent of students with perfect attendance were not statistically significant except for obese twelfth-grade girls, whose percentage was lower than all other fat classes. A similar situation, although not statistically significant, was apparent for eleventh-grade girls.

Lean boys tended to have fewer mean days of excused absences than did boys in other fat classes; for each of the three years they had a significantly lower mean than did average boys. Mean number of days of excused absences among girls' fat classes showed no significant differences except that in the eleventh and twelfth grades a higher percentage of obese girls had excused absences than did girls in other fat classes.

There were no consistent trends in mean number of days of unexcused absences among fat classes for either boys and girls, nor in percentages of each fat class having unexcused absences.

RACE. School attendance records classified by race (Table 6-XVIII) indicated that the Orientals had fewer absences than Caucasians and Negroes, and that there was a greater percentage of Orientals with perfect attendance.

In tenth, eleventh, and twelfth grades there was a significantly higher percentage of Oriental boys with perfect attendance than there were Caucasian and Negro boys. In eleventh grade the percentage of Caucasian boys with perfect attendance was significantly higher than that of the Negro boys.

Oriental boys also had a significantly lower number of excused absences than the other two races, and a lower percentage with such absences. Differences in mean days of excused absences and the percentage of each race having such absences were not significantly different between Caucasians and Negroes.

Unexcused absences followed the same pattern as excused absences for the Orientals. However, the Negro boys had a higher number of unexcused absences than the other two races, and a much higher percentage with such absences.

TABLE 6–XVIIA

SCHOOL ATTENDANCE RECORDS FOR TENTH-, ELEVENTH-, AND TWELFTH-GRADE STUDENTS CLASSIFIED BY PERCENT BODY FAT

Tenth Grade

FAT CLASSES	PERFECT ATTENDANCE	EXCUSED ABSENCES			UNEXCUSED ABSENCES			TOTAL N
	% Total Fat Class	$\bar{X}$ Days Absent	σ	% Total Fat Class	$\bar{X}$ Days Absent	σ	% Total Fat Class	
Boys								
Lean	19.0	4.1	3.69	78.6	2.0	2.49	23.8	42
Somewhat lean	24.2	4.6	4.36	71.0	2.8	1.71	19.4	62
Average	24.8	5.1	5.70	73.8	2.7	5.13	23.8	214
Somewhat obese	21.5	4.3	5.12	72.3	1.8	0.97	33.8	65
Obese	28.6	6.4	1.09	71.4	3.3	2.84	31.0	42
Girls								
Lean	14.3	4.1	3.54	85.7	2.6	1.67	9.6	42
Somewhat lean	21.9	4.8	4.66	73.4	3.1	5.73	18.8	64
Average	16.4	4.6	4.66	79.8	2.8	4.12	24.4	213
Somewhat obese	26.2	5.2	5.32	72.3	1.2	0.50	6.2	65
Obese	14.3	5.1	4.43	81.0	1.5	0.92	35.7	42

TABLE 6-XVIIB

SCHOOL ATTENDANCE RECORDS FOR TENTH-, ELEVENTH-, AND TWELFTH-GRADE STUDENTS CLASSIFIED BY PERCENT BODY FAT

Eleventh Grade

FAT CLASSES	PERFECT ATTENDANCE	EXCUSED ABSENCES			UNEXCUSED ABSENCES			TOTAL N
	% Total Fat Class	X̄ Days Absent	σ	% Total Fat Class	X̄ Days Absent	σ	% Total Fat Class	
Boys								
Lean	31.6	3.5	3.02	68.4	2.6	1.51	18.4	38
Somewhat lean	27.3	5.5	5.83	69.1	2.0	1.00	16.4	55
Average	28.2	4.5	4.26	67.6	3.0	2.82	25.0	188
Somewhat obese	29.1	4.6	4.69	70.9	3.6	3.38	23.6	55
Obese	35.9	4.6	6.46	64.1	2.7	1.15	7.7	39
Girls								
Lean	33.3	5.0	4.39	66.7	2.2	1.50	11.1	36
Somewhat lean	13.0	4.0	3.41	83.3	2.7	2.71	18.5	54
Average	18.1	5.0	4.31	80.1	1.5	0.83	19.3	171
Somewhat obese	18.9	5.2	5.40	81.1	2.1	1.64	20.8	53
Obese	6.1	5.4	5.20	90.9	7.2	13.17	18.2	33

TABLE 6–XVIIC

SCHOOL ATTENDANCE RECORDS FOR TENTH-, ELEVENTH-, AND TWELFTH-GRADE STUDENTS CLASSIFIED BY PERCENT BODY FAT

Twelfth Grade

FAT CLASSES	PERFECT ATTENDANCE	EXCUSED ABSENCES			UNEXCUSED ABSENCES			TOTAL N
	% Total Fat Class	$\bar{X}$ Days Absent	σ	% Total Fat Class	$\bar{X}$ Days Absent	σ	% Total Fat Class	
Boys								
Lean	13.2	4.1	3.47	81.6	1.7	2.10	28.9	38
Somewhat lean	21.4	5.3	4.90	76.8	3.3	3.63	32.1	56
Average	26.7	6.2	6.14	70.2	3.6	4.78	31.9	191
Somewhat obese	16.4	5.3	4.47	80.3	3.6	3.33	37.7	61
Obese	21.6	6.4	7.50	78.4	2.4	1.83	32.4	37
Girls								
Lean	20.5	5.1	3.76	76.9	4.9	4.13	25.6	39
Somewhat lean	20.3	5.1	5.20	72.9	2.0	1.58	35.6	59
Average	15.0	5.8	4.97	83.4	1.7	1.57	31.6	193
Somewhat obese	23.7	6.0	3.83	67.8	2.0	1.61	39.0	59
Obese	2.6	6.9	5.20	94.7	3.5	3.41	34.2	38

TABLE 6–XVIIIA

SCHOOL ATTENDANCE RECORDS FOR TENTH-, ELEVENTH-, AND TWELFTH-GRADE STUDENTS CLASSIFIED BY RACE

Tenth Grade

RACE	PERFECT ATTENDANCE	EXCUSED ABSENCES			UNEXCUSED ABSENCES			TOTAL N
	% Total Race	$\bar{X}$ Days Absent	σ	% Total Race	$\bar{X}$ Days Absent	σ	% Total Race	
Boys								
Caucasian	23.4	4.9	7.05	73.0	2.2	1.92	20.3	256
Negro	17.5	5.1	4.30	78.9	3.7	6.57	39.2	166
Oriental	42.5	3.4	2.83	57.5	1.5	1.00	10.0	40
Girls								
Caucasian	18.8	4.5	4.11	77.8	2.6	3.84	18.4	266
Negro	14.5	5.7	5.52	82.9	2.8	3.89	29.0	152
Oriental	29.7	2.8	2.46	64.9	1.0	0.00	8.1	37

TABLE 6–XVIIIB

SCHOOL ATTENDANCE RECORDS FOR TENTH-, ELEVENTH-, AND TWELFTH-GRADE STUDENTS
CLASSIFIED BY RACE

Eleventh Grade

RACE	PERFECT ATTENDANCE	EXCUSED ABSENCES			UNEXCUSED ABSENCES			TOTAL N
	% Total Race	X̄ Days Absent	σ	% Total Race	X̄ Days Absent	σ	% Total Race	
Boys								
Caucasian	28.9	4.9	5.06	67.1	4.6	6.14	19.7	249
Negro	16.5	5.7	5.92	79.1	3.5	3.23	39.2	158
Oriental	48.7	3.4	2.78	51.3	1.0 *	0.00	2.6	39
Girls								
Caucasian	15.3	5.6	5.03	82.3	2.2	1.56	17.7	249
Negro	14.6	6.1	5.65	84.7	3.1	5.34	30.6	144
Oriental	21.6	2.9	2.67	78.4	2.0 *	0.00	2.7	37

* N = 1.

TABLE 6-XVIIIC

SCHOOL ATTENDANCE RECORDS FOR TENTH-, ELEVENTH-, AND TWELFTH-GRADE STUDENTS
CLASSIFIED BY RACE

Twelfth Grade

RACE	PERFECT ATTENDANCE	EXCUSED ABSENCES			UNEXCUSED ABSENCES			TOTAL N
	% Total Race	X̄ Days Absent	σ	% Total Race	X̄ Days Absent	σ	% Total Race	
Boys								
Caucasian	22.0	6.2	6.51	74.8	3.0	3.83	28.3	254
Negro	16.0	5.8	5.52	78.2	4.3	5.04	46.8	156
Oriental	51.3	3.8	2.94	46.2	1.2	0.45	12.8	39
Girls								
Caucasian	17.8	5.8	4.92	79.7	2.4	2.59	26.6	241
Negro	8.1	7.0	5.37	87.9	2.2	2.10	50.8	124
Oriental	40.0	2.6	2.48	60.0	1.0	0.00	8.6	35

The percentage of Oriental girls with perfect attendance was significantly higher than that of the Negro girls in tenth and twelfth grades, and higher than the Caucasians in twelfth grade. There was a significantly higher percentage of Caucasian girls with perfect attendance in the twelfth grade than Negro girls.

Again, Oriental girls had a lower mean number of excused absences than the other two races for all three grades. The percentage of Oriental girls having these absences was slightly lower than the percentages for Caucasians and Negroes. In tenth and twelfth grades, Negro girls had a significantly higher mean number of excused absences than Caucasians, but the percentages of each race having such absences was quite similar.

There were no statistically significant racial differences among the girls in mean number of unexcused absences, although the Oriental mean was lower than that of the other two races in each grade. A more pronounced difference was observed in the percentage of each race having unexcused absences; the Orientals had the lowest percentage, the Caucasians the next lowest, and the Negroes the highest.

SOCIOECONOMIC LEVEL. The boys in the lower-third socioeconomic level had a significantly lower percentage with perfect attendance records than did boys in the higher levels in tenth and eleventh grades, but not in twelfth grade (Table 6-XIX).

The mean days of excused absences did not differ significantly among the levels; however, there was a trend for the middle-third level to have more days of excused absences, the upper-third the least. The lower-third group had a greater percentage of its members with excused absences in all grades except the twelfth, when percentages were equal for all levels.

The percentage of upper-third boys with unexcused absences was lower than the other levels all three years, while lower-third boys had a higher percentage in tenth and eleventh grades than the other levels. In twelfth grade the lower- and middle-third groups were equal in the percentage of their members who had unexcused absences. Mean number of days of unexcused absences for the three levels did not repeat these trends.

Perfect attendance percentages among girls in the three

TABLE 6-XIXA

SCHOOL ATTENDANCE RECORDS FOR TENTH-, ELEVENTH-, AND TWELFTH-GRADE STUDENTS CLASSIFIED BY SOCIOECONOMIC LEVEL

Tenth Grade

SOCIO-ECONOMIC LEVEL	PERFECT ATTENDANCE % Total Level	EXCUSED ABSENCES			UNEXCUSED ABSENCES			TOTAL N
		X̄ Days Absent	σ	% Total Level	X̄ Days Absent	σ	% Total Level	
Boys								
Lower-third	9.3	4.0	2.43	88.4	4.1	8.59	37.2	43
Middle-third	30.7	4.5	4.11	67.8	2.0	1.36	17.6	199
Upper-third	28.1	3.4	2.60	71.1	2.1	1.71	11.4	114
Girls								
Lower-third	13.9	6.1	5.64	83.3	2.1	1.24	33.3	36
Middle-third	19.4	4.5	4.03	78.1	1.9	2.05	16.3	196
Upper-third	20.0	3.7	2.92	77.5	2.6	4.77	16.7	120

TABLE 6–XIXB

SCHOOL ATTENDANCE RECORDS FOR TENTH-, ELEVENTH-, AND TWELFTH-GRADE STUDENTS CLASSIFIED BY SOCIOECONOMIC LEVEL

Eleventh Grade

SOCIO-ECONOMIC LEVEL	PERFECT ATTENDANCE	EXCUSED ABSENCES			UNEXCUSED ABSENCES			TOTAL N
	% Total Level	X̄ Days Absent	σ	% Total Level	X̄ Days Absent	σ	% Total Level	
Boys								
Lower-third	10.2	4.3	4.00	89.8	3.6	3.82	34.7	49
Middle-third	31.4	5.1	5.06	66.2	3.2	2.42	22.5	204
Upper-third	34.2	3.8	4.49	61.5	1.5	0.65	12.0	117
Girls								
Lower-third	20.0	5.1	3.68	80.0	1.6	1.03	31.4	35
Middle-third	19.8	5.0	4.46	78.1	2.8	5.60	18.8	192
Upper-third	13.4	4.8	4.71	84.9	2.1	1.32	15.1	119

TABLE 6–XIXC

SCHOOL ATTENDANCE RECORDS FOR TENTH-, ELEVENTH-, AND TWELFTH-GRADE STUDENTS CLASSIFIED BY SOCIOECONOMIC LEVEL

Twelfth Grade

SOCIO-ECONOMIC LEVEL	PERFECT ATTENDANCE	EXCUSED ABSENCES			UNEXCUSED ABSENCES			TOTAL N
	% Total Level	$\bar{X}$ Days Absent	σ	% Total Level	$\bar{X}$ Days Absent	σ	% Total Level	
Boys								
Lower-third	19.4	6.0	5.08	74.2	4.2	4.97	38.7	62
Middle-third	22.3	6.2	6.33	73.1	3.2	3.80	38.2	238
Upper-third	25.6	5.2	5.03	73.7	4.4	6.85	23.7	156
Girls								
Lower-third	10.4	7.8	5.95	89.6	2.6	2.79	47.9	48
Middle-third	16.1	5.9	4.91	81.0	2.2	1.77	31.3	211
Upper-third	19.4	5.1	4.24	77.0	2.3	2.80	30.9	139

socioeconomic levels did not show any significant differences or trends.

Mean number of days of excused absences were significantly higher for girls in the lower-third group than for the other two levels in tenth and twelfth grades. No socioeconomic differences appeared in percentage of girls in each level with excused absences.

The percentage of girls with unexcused absences was higher in the lower-third level than in the other levels all three years. No trends were found in mean number of unexcused absences.

Summary

Obese boys and girls tended to do less well than other body fat classes in physical performance test scores. There were no clear-cut racial trends in the physical performance test scores for either sex.

Obese teenagers tended to have grades lower than others. Oriental teenagers tended to have higher grades and Negroes lower grades than did Caucasians. Teenagers in the lower socio-economic level had lower grades than those in the middle and upper levels.

School attendance did not seem related to body fat. Orientals had better attendance records than Caucasians or Negroes. The school attendance of those in the lower socioeconomic class was poorer than that of teenagers in the middle or upper classes.

CHAPTER 7

TEENAGERS' ATTITUDES*

O NE OF THE LONG-TERM GOALS of this study was to apply the findings in a coordinated community program promoting physical fitness and weight control, i.e. prevention or reversal of obesity or extreme leanness. Since this kind of educational effort would be directed toward behavioral change, it would need to be built on any interest the teenager might have in physical fitness, weight control, and body conformation. For this reason, questionnaires were used to investigate their interest in these matters.

This chapter reports some of our findings over a four-year period from the questionnaires concerning teenagers' own views on eating practices, activity, and body composition and conformation. The questions were oriented toward practical nutrition and activity programming. Students' replies were accepted at face value. Although our observations led to some speculation, we did not attempt to probe into possible psychological reasons that might have prompted students to answer as they did. We explored statistical associations between replies and gross body composition wherever they appeared to be meaningful.

Table 2-I indicates numbers of subjects who answered questionnaires each year. Race and body fat were not known for all subjects who answered questionnaires. Although Oriental subjects were too few to constitute a significant group, some of their responses will be mentioned for the trends they suggest. The percentage of boys and girls in the total sample and in the longitudinal sample giving similar replies to each of the repeated questions were compared. For no reply category did these per-

* The substance of this chapter appeared originally in *The American Journal of Clinical Nutrition, 18:325*, May 1966, to which we are indebted for its use.

centages differ by more than 6 percent, and in all instances changes over time were equally apparent in either set of data. Since the results were virtually the same whether based on the longitudinal or total sample, only the data derived from the total sample are reported in detail.

Food and Eating Practices

Meal Preference

The opening question, "Which meal do you like best?" was of low emotional tone to allay the subjects' possible resentment toward being questioned about eating practices; nevertheless, it yielded results that might be of practical value. Table 7-I shows that dinner was the preferred meal, especially for boys. Conversely, more girls than boys chose lunch. Breakfast was almost as popular as lunch with the boys, but not so with the girls.

Race also appeared to influence choices, as shown in Table

TABLE 7–I

REPLIES OF NINTH- AND ELEVENTH-GRADE STUDENTS
CLASSIFIED BY RACE TO: "WHICH MEAL DO YOU LIKE BEST?"

Replies	Caucasian %	Negro %	Oriental %	All %
Ninth-grade boys				
Breakfast	9.3	4.9	10.6	8.4
Lunch	9.7	8.2	4.2	9.0
Dinner	74.8	64.8	74.5	70.8
Other responses	6.2	22.1	10.7	9.8
Ninth-grade girls				
Breakfast	9.1	6.5	2.6	7.3
Lunch	19.7	14.4	7.7	17.5
Dinner	65.0	50.4	79.5	61.5
Other responses	6.2	28.7	10.2	11.7
Eleventh-grade boys				
Breakfast	7.6	11.1	8.6	9.0
Lunch	8.0	6.9	5.7	7.3
Dinner	80.2	74.3	85.7	78.7
Other responses	4.2	7.7	0.0	4.7
Eleventh-grade girls				
Breakfast	7.7	8.6	8.3	8.5
Lunch	11.4	18.6	2.8	13.0
Dinner	76.8	64.3	86.1	73.2
Other responses	4.1	8.5	2.8	4.9

7-I. In the ninth grade a statistically significant difference appeared between Negro and Caucasian boys in dinner choice; differences were insignificant in the eleventh grade. At both grade levels, Negro girls' choice of dinner ranked significantly lower than that of girls of other races.

That this racial difference may have had a socioeconomic component was implied at the ninth-grade level when students were attending three different schools. There was a significantly higher dinner preference in School "C," of relatively high socioeconomic status, than in Schools "A" and "B." School C was predominantly Caucasian, with too few Negro and Oriental students to permit statistically valid racial comparison with other schools. The tendency for dinner to be more popular with the upper-middle-class Caucasian group may have practical implications for the teaching of nutrition.

Significant associations between body composition and meal preference were found only in the ninth grade. Lean boys showed the lowest (60 percent) and obese boys the highest (92 percent) level of dinner preference. Interestingly, for the girls the reverse situation held, with 80 percent of the lean and only 56 percent of the obese favoring this meal. Were some of the obese girls perhaps reluctant to express a liking for the big meal of the day?

The reasons stated for meal preferences give some indication of teenage values. Table 7-II summarizes the leading responses. It is interesting to note that while ninth-grade boys and girls were alike in stating the type of food served as the most frequent reason for their choice, the less frequent reasons of variety in food and company present were mentioned much oftener by girls than boys. By the eleventh grade, environment seemed to have become more important to both sexes and type of food less so.

Between the ninth- and eleventh-grade levels, we noted some difference among races in the order of frequency of the above replies. As ninth graders, Oriental children led other races in the proportion mentioning surroundings and eating with family. At both grade levels the Negro children, on the other hand, mentioned nutrition and health reasons more often than did other races.

TABLE 7–II

PERCENT OF NINTH- AND ELEVENTH-GRADE STUDENTS STATING
SPECIFIED REASONS FOR MEAL PREFERENCES

| | Ninth Grade | | Eleventh Grade | |
	Boys (N = 465) %	Girls (N = 519) %	Boys (N = 426) %	Girls (N = 425) %
Type of food	31	34	11	15
Large amount of food	23	9	30	13
Relief from hunger, tiredness, "growling stomach," etc.	16	13	21	20
Environment at meal time: "I can eat leisurely," "I can watch TV," "I like the surroundings," etc.	12	13	19	32
Variety: "many dishes," "each meal different," etc.	7	13	7	12
Company present: family, friends	6	19	3	12
Healthful effect: "It is well balanced," "It builds me up," "It supplies vitamins," etc.	9	9	7	14

The only reason significantly associated with body composition was that of "large amount of food," mentioned by a greater proportion of the lean ninth-grade girls.

Viewing reasons for meal preference in association with the specific meal chosen, we found results that may have practical implications. At both grade levels leading reasons stated by those who preferred breakfast were its effect in providing energy ("It peps me up," "It keeps me going until lunch," etc.) and relief from hunger. Thus, its chief appeal lay in its effect rather than in the meal itself.

The three leading reasons for choosing lunch in both ninth and eleventh grades were the company of friends, the freedom experienced at this meal, and relief from hunger. It appears, therefore, that social factors should be considered when planning lunches for students.

In the case of dinner, about 70 percent of the ninth and eleventh graders who chose this meal as their favorite gave food as the reason: the type, the amount, the method of preparation and the wide variety offered. Second in frequency, but totaling only about 17 percent for boys and 38 percent for girls, were reasons related to the atmosphere at dinner time (feelings of leisure, surroundings, etc.). Hunger ranked third, and company present fourth. Thus, to please teenagers with a dinner, it would appear important to pay particular attention to the food itself.

Ideas on Who Knows Good-tasting Food

Since food is an important factor influencing teenagers' meal preferences, whose food tastes do they emulate? Table 7-III gives responses to the question, "In your opinion, which person in your family or among your friends has the best ideas about good-tasting foods?" In line with the finding of Litman, Cooney and Stief (1964), that the mother was the authority figure for their

TABLE 7-III

REPLIES OF NINTH- AND ELEVENTH-GRADERS TO:
"WHO HAS THE BEST IDEA ABOUT GOOD-TASTING FOODS?"

| | Boys | | Girls | |
| | 9th Grade (N = 438) | 11th Grade (N = 426) | 9th Grade (N = 500) | 11th Grade (N = 425) |
Replies	%	%	%	%
Father	16.3	16.2	11.2	12.9
Mother	35.7	39.4	45.7	52.9
Mother and father	3.9	2.8	3.1	2.6
Sibling	11.0	8.9	8.3	6.4
Other relative	5.0	3.8	4.8	2.6
Other adult	0.4	1.2	2.1	1.2
Teenage friend	3.0	2.6	3.7	5.4
Self	13.3	14.5	7.9	9.9
Mother and other females	1.7	0.7	2.9	0.5
Father and other males	0.2	0.0	0.2	0.0
No answer	9.5	9.9	10.2	5.6

subjects (whose ages were from ten to 22), our results from ninth graders showed that parents definitely outranked peers as food authorities.

We found no associations that were statistically significant between replies indicating food authorities and race, school attended, or body composition.

TABLE 7–IV

NINTH- AND ELEVENTH-GRADE REPLIES TO:
"WHAT FOODS SHOULD BE EATEN EVERY DAY FOR HEALTH?"

| | Boys | | Girls | |
| | 9th Grade (N = 465) % | 11th Grade (N = 426) % | 9th Grade (N = 519) % | 11th Grade (N = 425) % |
Replies				
Milk	66.5	69.0	76.7	82.8
Meat	81.5	84.5	86.3	93.2
Fruits/Vegetables	83.4	84.3	90.2	94.6
Grain foods	35.9	42.5	56.1	58.6
Sugar foods	9.5	9.4	10.0	10.8
Fats	5.8	4.0	6.7	3.8
Liquid	6.7	4.9	6.4	4.7
Vitamin supplement	0.6	2.4	0.6	1.4

Concept of Healthful Foods

Because some studies (Hinton *et al.,* 1963; Young, Berresford and Waldner, 1956) have found knowledge of nutrition positively related to good food practices, we asked the question, "What foods should be eaten every day for health?" It was asked in these terms to relate it to popular nutrition teaching. For the same reason, we evaluated replies using the "Basic Four" (U.S.D.A., 1958) food groups. Table 7-IV summarizes the replies. Contrary to our expectations, fruits and vegetables, and also meat, were mentioned more frequently than milk by both boys and girls. Cereal grain foods were not commonly considered essential. The teenagers' frequent mention of items such as sugar, liquids, fats, and vitamin supplements suggests that a number of students may have been somewhat confused by what they had heard from one source or another. About half of the subjects in both years mentioned all four of the basic food groups. The results indicate, therefore, that knowledge of these food groups had reached many of the students.

Fewer boys than girls included each of the four food groups in their replies. The only racial difference was that in the eleventh grade more Caucasian and Oriental than Negro boys mentioned milk, meat, and vegetables. In the ninth grade, when students were in separate schools, those from the school of highest socioeconomic level listed each of the "Basic Four" food groups with greatest frequency.

Opinions About Taking Vitamin Supplements. Because some students in both the ninth and eleventh grades had voluntarily listed "vitamin pills" with foods they considered essential for health, we included the specific question, "What do you think of a high school student's taking a daily vitamin pill?" in the questionnaire administered in the tenth and twelfth grades. Replies are summarized in Figure 7–1.

Opinions of Their Own Diets. Table 7-V showing ninth-grade students' ratings of the healthfulness of their own diets indicates that they did not agree with the commonly held poor

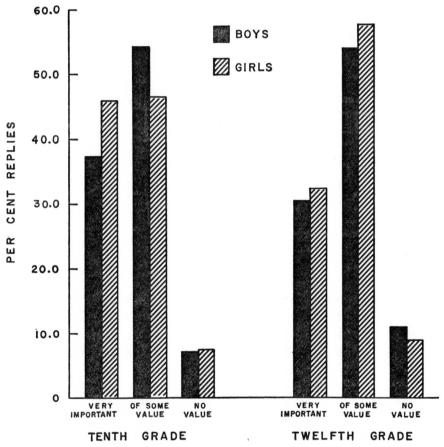

Figure 7–1. Replies of tenth- and twelfth-grade students to: "What do you think of a high school student taking a daily vitamin pill?"

opinion of teenage diets. We found that sex, race, body composition, and socioeconomic status were not significantly associated with these diet ratings.

Do students base their judgment of their own diet on some knowledge of what foods may constitute dietary adequacy? We compared students' self-ratings with their answers to the question, "What foods should be eaten every day for health?" and found that of those who had rated their diets as "excellent," 66 percent had mentioned milk, 84 percent fruits and vegetables, 83 percent meats, and 43 percent cereals. We cannot say, therefore, that all ratings of "excellent" were made with the "Basic Four" food groups in mind.

Comparisons with actual intake as shown by dietary records are presented in Chapter 4.

TABLE 7–V

REPLIES OF NINTH-GRADE STUDENTS TO:
"HOW WOULD YOU GRADE THE
HEALTHFULNESS OF WHAT YOU EAT?"

	Boys N = 465 %	*Girls* N = 519 %
Poor	2.2	2.3
Fair	25.8	28.7
Good	51.2	55.5
Excellent	20.0	12.9
No answer	0.8	0.6

Opinions of Teenage Food Practices

To augment the earlier question regarding students' opinions of their own diets, we asked the ninth grade a final question about food practices, primarily to arouse reactions and discussion. It was the obviously provocative question, "Some people say teenagers don't eat the right foods. Do you agree with the people who say this? Why do you agree or disagree?"

Approximately 44 percent of the boys and 48 percent of the girls said they agreed with the statement, while 3 percent and 5 percent respectively said that food choices were "sometimes right and sometimes wrong," and most of the rest disagreed.

The reasons for disagreeing included such statements as

"teenagers eat as well as adults" and "people's views on teenagers' eating habits are inaccurate, prejudiced, or overgeneralized," while others commented that teenagers eat well because "parents provide good guidance." Recognition of parental guidance in eating has been mentioned in other studies (Litman, Cooney and Stief, 1964). Those who agreed with the indictment of teenage diets mentioned such factors as time pressures, the peer-group influence, and poor motivation. Only three people mentioned the school cafeteria; one girl said it was helpful and two boys said it was not.

The relationship between students' degree of fatness or leanness and their opinion of teenage eating practices was examined. The leanest students, especially the girls, tended to be more critical of teenage eating practices than the obese.

Frequency of Hunger

Feelings of hunger may well influence not only the quantity and type of food eaten, but also when and how often it is eaten. That these factors may be associated with body composition is indicated by Stunkard's finding (Stunkard, Grace and Wolff, 1955) that the "night eating syndrome" was characteristic of the obese. Likewise the popular stereotype of the lean teenage boy as being always hungry and the lean girl as being a finicky eater imply an association. Does such a relationship exist in this group of students? We asked them to indicate on a five-point scale how often they were hungry ("all the time," "most of the time," "some of the time" "hardly ever," "never"), and also to indicate on a time line the approximate times of day they were usually most hungry.

Table 7-VI shows the frequency of hunger of students classified by sex and body fat. The greatest percentage of both boys and girls fell into the "some of the time" category, and the smallest percentage into the "hardly ever" or "never" class. There was, however, a smaller percentage of boys than girls in the latter category. Conversely, there was a significantly higher percentage of boys than girls in the "all" or "most of the time" classes. These comparisons between the sexes held for all classifications of body fat.

TABLE 7–VI

FREQUENCY OF HUNGER IN PERCENT OF NINTH-GRADE
STUDENTS CLASSIFIED BY SEX AND BODY FAT

	"All" or "Most of the time" %	"Some of the time" %	"Hardly ever" or "Never" %	No Answer %	N
Boys					
Lean	48.8	46.5	4.7	0.0	43
Somewhat lean	58.1	38.7	3.2	0.0	62
Average	42.8	50.2	7.0	0.0	201
Somewhat obese	41.4	48.3	10.3	0.0	58
Obese	43.6	56.4	0.0	0.0	39
Total boys	46.9	48.1	5.0	0.0	403
Girls					
Lean	34.0	56.0	10.0	0.0	50
Somewhat lean	48.0	48.0	4.0	0.0	75
Average	32.8	53.5	13.3	0.4	241
Somewhat obese	27.8	61.1	11.1	0.0	72
Obese	25.0	62.5	10.4	2.1	48
Total girls	33.5	56.2	9.8	0.5	486

Eppright, Sidwell and Swanson (1954) found a decrease in caloric intake of girls at this age level, possibly due to lessened needs. Also, Hinton and associates (1963) found that fat girls of this age group "were inclined to enjoy food less." Were the girls in our study really less hungry than the boys or did they feel it was culturally unacceptable to admit being hungry?

We found socioeconomic factors, measured by school attended, not significantly associated with frequency of hunger.

When students were asked to indicate on a time line extending from "earlier than 6:00 A.M." to "later than 9.00 P.M." the time of day when they were usually most hungry, 12:00 noon and 6:00 P.M. received the greatest number of checks. The time most frequently checked by the girls was 12:00 noon, while the boys checked 12:00 noon and 6:00 P.M. with equal frequency. There was no indication that those in the obese and somewhat obese groups tended to be hungry later in the day, as might have occurred in the "night eating syndrome" of Stunkard (1955). The small number of checks before 8:00 A.M. tended to verify our previously mentioned finding that breakfast was not a favorite meal.

Questions regarding frequency of hunger were not repeated in the eleventh grade.

How the Teenager Views His Own Figure

The popular impression that teenagers growing into young men and women are keenly interested in the size and shape of their developing figures was well documented by their responses to the questionnaires. The teenagers' predominant attitude was dissatisfaction—with their weight, fatness or leanness, stature, and certain other body dimensions. The girls' self-perception regarding fatness and leanness was in sharp contrast to that of the boys. Large numbers of girls described themselves as fat, the numbers increasing from 43 percent in the ninth grade to 56 percent in the twelfth grade. Most boys either thought they were too thin or seemed satisfied with their body conformation. More than 50 percent of the girls said they were "extremely" or "fairly" concerned about overweight, matching almost identically the boys' expressed concern about underweight. That weight was much more of a problem to girls than to boys bears out Deischer's observations in surveying the health concerns of adolescents aged twelve to eighteen years (Deischer and Mills, 1963).

Differences in attitudes toward their own body size and conformation were discernible among the three races. For both sexes, Caucasians and Orientals were more likely than Negroes to think themselves fat from ninth to twelfth grade. Negro boys and girls tended to consider themselves "about right" or a little too thin, but there was a steady increase, as time passed, in the numbers of Negro girls who thought themselves fat. Although underweight was a relatively low priority concern for any of the girls, more Negro girls said they were concerned about underweight than did Caucasian girls. Oriental girls in twelfth grade surpassed all others in their self-perception of fatness and in concerns about both overweight and underweight. Almost twice as many Negro as Caucasian boys (65 percent versus 35 percent) indicated concern about underweight.

How did this compare with their fatness as determined anthropometrically? In grades ten and twelve over half the Caucasian girls called themselves fat in some degree, while only a fourth of them were classed as obese or somewhat obese on the basis of measurements. The Oriental girls differed even more than did the Caucasians in this respect. However, the group of Negro girls who considered themselves obese was only a few percentage points greater than the group who actually were obese.

STATURE AND BODY DIMENSIONS. As shown in Figure 7–2 boys generally wanted to be taller in both tenth and twelfth grades, while girls seemed content with their stature.

Half or more of all boys in tenth and twelfth grades expressed a desire for larger biceps, chest, wrists, shoulders, and/or forearms, with the wish for a change in biceps outranking all others. Negro boys in tenth and twelfth grades seemed more eager than the others for increases in all body dimensions. One-fourth or more specified wanting, in addition to those areas listed above, larger waists, hips, thighs, calves, and ankles. They appeared simply to want to be bigger.

Half or more of all girls said they wanted smaller hip, thigh, and/or waist measurements, in that rank order. Negro girls seemed more satisfied with their figures than did Caucasians. Almost twice the percentage of tenth- and twelfth-grade Caucasian as Negro girls wished for smaller hips and thighs. Smaller waists had priority over smaller thighs for Negro girls, and one-fifth or more said they wanted larger hips and/or thighs. Measurements of the girls revealed that the Negro tenth-grade girls had average waist and hip measurements similar to those of Caucasian girls. Two years later they were larger than Caucasians in these dimensions, but apparently this did not interfere with their desire for increases or for no change at all. The ideal figure, it appears, is not the same for Negro and Caucasian girls.

SELF-DESCRIPTION VERSUS ACTUAL MEASUREMENTS. How realistically did the subjects view themselves? The obese group appeared to acknowledge their obesity. Of the 39 boys and 48 girls in the ninth grade who were classified as obese all but seven and six, respectively, described themselves as overweight. In the twelfth grade all but two of the obese boys and two of the obese girls so described themselves, and a great majority said they wished to lose weight.

However, when we consider the total group of subjects and compare their expressed desire to gain or lose weight with their

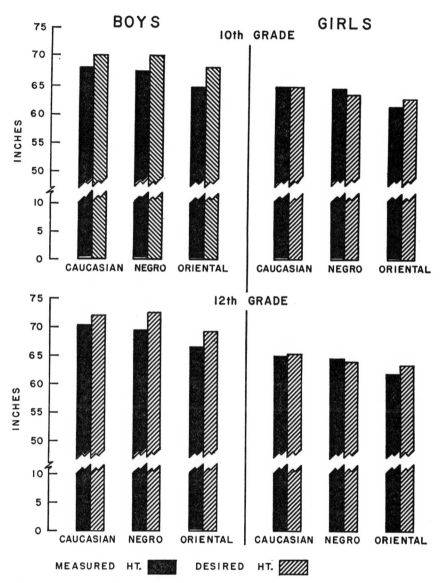

Figure 7–2. Comparison of mean heights, measured and desired, of tenth- and twelfth-grade boys and girls, by race.

body fat as determined anthropometrically, many seem to have unrealistic self-images not in keeping with their objective measurements. Sixty-three percent of all ninth-grade girls wanted to lose weight, and so did 70 percent of tenth- and twelfth-grade girls. These numbers far exceed the numbers who described themselves as fat and indicated concern about overweight. They also contrast sharply with the 15 percent and 10 percent which each year we arbitrarily classified as the somewhat obese and obese groups, respectively.

Nor were the boys much more realistic in their fervor for weight gain. Fifty-three percent of the ninth-grade boys and 59 percent of the tenth- and twelfth-grade boys said they wanted to gain weight, many more than described themselves as thin and said they were concerned about underweight. These figures too, contrast sharply with the 25 percent each year whose anthropometric evaluation classified them as lower than average in fatness. We speculate that the boys who considered themselves too thin and wanted to gain weight were not interested in gaining weight *per se* but rather in becoming more muscular, and equated this with added weight. The measurements they thought to be too small are muscular—biceps and forearm, or areas which when well-developed are popularly considered to be associated with masculinity—chest and shoulders.

Weight Control Efforts

Had their concern about weight motivated the teenagers into any course of action? In the ninth grade 50 percent of the boys and 65 percent of the girls said they were trying to do *something* about their weight.

Changes in diet outranked changes in physical activity as chosen methods of weight control. For each ninth-grade boy who mentioned exercise as a means of adjusting weight, one and one-third mentioned diet. For each girl who listed exercise, two and one-half specified diet. Limiting amount or kind of food as a weight control method was mentioned by three girls to each boy.

An acknowledged effort to control weight had tapered off by the twelfth grade to 34 percent of the boys and 55 percent of the girls. The ratio of diet to exercise was now one to one for the boys, still two and a half to one for the girls, and five girls to one boy mentioned limiting food intake.

WEIGHT CONTROL EFFORTS AS AFFECTED BY BODY COMPOSITION. More obese boys than their leaner classmates indicated trying to do something about weight in grades nine and twelve. In both years the obese boys said they were limiting food far more than this was reported by others. Also, more of them said they were exercising.

Similarly, obese girls in grades nine and twelve exceeded all other girls in claiming action about their weight. Both the obese and somewhat obese surpassed by far the other girls who said they were limiting food, especially in the twelfth grade. The somewhat obese girls reported exercising more than others, with the obese girls in second place.

WEIGHT CONTROL EFFORTS AS AFFECTED BY RACE. Action for weight control also varied by racial groups. A greater percent of the Negro boys said they were trying to gain weight or size. Of the boys whose stated desire was to lose weight or size, the Caucasian boys indicated limiting their food intake and exercising more often than the Negro boys did. Between ninth and twelfth grades there was an increase in Caucasian and a decrease in Negro boys who answered affirmatively the question, "Are you trying to do anything about your weight?" Almost twice as many Caucasians as Negroes said "Yes."

In the twelfth grade, although a smaller percent of Orientals than Caucasians said they were doing something about their weight, they were likely to be eating and exercising more than were the Caucasian boys, to achieve their goals of weight gain and increase in size.

About two-thirds of the girls in all racial groups said they were trying to do something about their weight in the ninth grade. More Caucasians than Negroes said they were modifying their diet—eating either more or less—to adjust their weight. Also, the Caucasian girls mentioned exercise as a chosen method of weight control four times as often as the Negro girls. The Oriental girls in the ninth grade fell between Negro and Caucasian

TABLE 7–VII

RESULTS OF WEIGHT REDUCTION EFFORTS

Questionnaire Responses	Boys N	Girls N
In ninth grade, reported dieting to lose weight	26	91
Had less body fat in twelfth grade (5 * to 18 percentage points)	5	14
Had more body fat in twelfth grade (5 * to 12 percentage points)	3	14
Had same * percentage of body fat in twelfth grade	18	63
In twelfth grade still trying to lose weight by "dieting"	15	69

* Changes of less than five percentage points were arbitrarily considered to be within the range of normal daily weight change and/or measurement error. Thus lesser fat changes are not considered significant.

girls in these actions. By grade twelve, when interest in weight control had waned somewhat for all girls, these racial differences remained the same.

RESULTS OF WEIGHT REDUCTION EFFORTS. Having revealed in the ninth grade dissatisfaction with their body size and shape of sufficient magnitude to encourage changes in their eating and exercise patterns, what results did they achieve? Table 7-VII shows that about one out of five boys and one out of six girls

TABLE 7–VIII

NINTH- AND TWELFTH-GRADE REPLIES TO: "IF A PERSON IS FAT, WHAT IS MOST LIKELY TO BE THE REASON?"

Questionnaire Responses *	Boys		Girls	
	Ninth Grade (N = 465) %	Twelfth Grade (N = 460) %	Ninth Grade (N = 519) %	Twelfth Grade (N = 379) %
He eats too much.**	56	42	64	63
He doesn't exercise enough.**	48	46	42	42
It is natural for him to be fat.**	23	25	19	12
Glands	4	3	6	6
Psychological problems	3	2	6	4
He eats wrong foods.	2	<1	4	3

* Multiple responses given.
** Itemized in check list.

did succeed in reducing body fat from the ninth to the twelfth grade. Almost an equal number had gained fat, however.

Knowledge of the Causes of Obesity

Considering their preoccupations with obesity, real or imagined, and their efforts to do something about it, what understanding did the students have of the causes of obesity? By the ninth grade most of them seemed, indeed, to be aware of the principal factors involved in obesity (Table 7-VIII), although popular misconceptions were evident.

Attitudes Toward Dietary Changes

The focus of the questionnaires used in tenth and twelfth grades shifted from *what* the subjects were attempting to do about their weight to *how they felt* about certain diet and exercise measures for changing body shape and size. The responses concerning diet differed distinctly according to sex. Girls seemed generally more accepting than boys of dietary modifications.

LIQUID FORMULAS. Although a majority of tenth-grade boys (77 percent) and girls (60 percent) disapproved of liquid formula diets, a sizeable minority (21 percent and 37 percent respectively) favored their use as a substitute for one meal a day. Between tenth and twelfth grades the changes in responses shifted from disapproval to approval.

MILK. Approximately two-thirds of the girls but fewer than half of the boys said they favored the use of skim instead of whole milk. The Negro boys in both years objected more than the Caucasians to the skim milk.

Negro girls were far less accepting of skim milk in both years than were Caucasians and Orientals, almost half of them disapproving as compared with three-fourths of Caucasians and Orientals who favored it.

FATS. The majority of both boys and girls said they would be willing to reduce dietary fat such as mayonnaise, french fries, bacon, etc.

FRUITS AND VEGETABLES. Because weight control diets are likely to emphasize fruits and vegetables the students were asked to rate their willingness to eat extra amounts of these foods. An overwhelming majority of boys and girls, especially the latter, indicated fair to good acceptance of both. Fruit received more approval than vegetables by both sexes and all racial groups. Obese boys tended to give a higher rating than other boys did to extra fruit, and tenth-grade obese girls tended to greater willingness than other girls for extra vegetables.

SWEETS. Students were then asked to assume that they were overweight and to rate their willingness to eliminate almost all sweets from their own diet as a means of reducing. In both tenth and twelfth grades 66 percent of the boys and 79 percent of the girls indicated willingness to do this.

Attitudes Toward Physical Activity

Students were asked to rate various types of physical activity in the question: "If you had to advise a person like yourself on a plan to develop a good figure, how would you rate these methods of exercise: calisthenics, strenuous work, recreational exercise, walking, and competitive sports?" Appropriate examples were given to assist in making choices. Responses of the tenth-grade boys show calisthenics, recreational exercise, and competitive sports almost equally high choices. Ratings were similar in the twelfth grade, except that recreational exercise dropped below the other two. For girls in tenth and twelfth grades, recreational exercise was clearly the first choice, followed by walking, calisthenics, and competitive sports in descending order. Although strenuous work was at the bottom of the list for girls, 40 percent of the boys rated it high. High rating for strenuous work is of particular interest, because around-the-clock activity diaries recorded by a subsample of students for four one-week periods (reported in Chapter 5) revealed that these boys and girls had barely a nodding acquaintance with strenuous work.

Racial and grade level differences were minor, except that Negro girls in twelfth grade rated competitive sports higher and walking lower than Caucasian girls did.

Conclusions

The majority of both sexes, all races, and all body composition groupings expressed willingness to do something about their size, shape, and fatness or leanness—the boys tending to choose exercise more often than the girls. Many said they actually were trying to do something about their weight. Among those who reported modifying their diet to lose weight, few had succeeded. Majority opinions revealed that dinner was the favorite meal and that parents were acknowledged as leading food authorities. Most teenagers rated their own diets as fair or better, although only about half of them mentioned all four basic food groups. In general, these teenagers had a reasonably good knowledge of dietary needs and causes of obesity, although some had misconceptions. Some differences among races and among socioeconomic levels were revealed in concepts of desirable body conformation, in choice of diet, and in favorite patterns of physical activity.

Summary

A series of four questionnaires was administered to subjects, one each year from ninth to twelfth grades. The purpose was to investigate teenagers' views on their own body size and shape, their eating practices, their activities, and their interest and action in modifying any of these. Some questions were repeated in another year to see if changes had occurred.

Responses indicated that these teenagers had a high degree of interest in their body conformation, sustained from the ninth to twelfth grade, and that they were generally dissatisfied with their size and shape. Boys' desires were mainly to gain weight and/or size, girls' to lose weight and reduce certain dimensions. Boys were more favorable to exercise for figure development, girls to diet. The majority of both sexes, all racial groups, and all body fat classes (lean to obese) were willing, they said, to carry out action programs for figure change. Of those who had already changed their diet for weight reduction, few had succeeded in three years, and the remainder were as likely to have gained weight as to have lost it.

Many of the teenagers revealed unrealistic views of their fatness or leanness, mainly Caucasian girls whose evaluation of their own excessive fatness differed considerably from their actual measurements.

Racial differences were noted in concepts of ideal body size and shape, in choice of diet, in meal preference, and in types of activities favored.

The information yielded will be valuable in planning and implementing a community program promoting weight control and physical fitness.

CHAPTER 8

IMPLICATIONS

THIS CHAPTER IS TO HIGHLIGHT findings which we believe have implications for future studies and for planning public health programs.

BODY MEASUREMENTS. The need for developing and testing a practical method of assessing gross body composition was one of the reasons for initiating this study. Inadequacies of height and weight measurements only and the impracticality of body density determinations for routine use in public schools, clinics or private physicians' offices have been previously discussed (Chapter 3). The Behnke body envelope method was found to yield results compatible with those resulting from use of the more involved body density and K_{40} determinations (Table 3-IV). The measurements themselves did not require an undue amount of time, and the method was easily learned. In order to reduce measuring time to a minimum, two methods using a smaller number of measurements were developed (Appendix A). The calculations are not time-consuming when done by computer. We believe therefore that a system for determining gross body composition by utilizing a limited number of body circumferences and diameters is feasible for use in schools. Such a practical method is essential to a surveillance program aimed at obesity prevention.

Our finding that 70 percent of the girls wanted to lose weight regardless of their body composition indicates that students, especially girls, need to learn more realistic norms for body weight. Routine assessment of gross body composition could teach students a more rational standard and tend to motivate them to control their weight. Systematic assessment, even of height and weight only, in schools not yet able to do computer analyses could do much toward alerting students to the importance of maintaining control of their weight.

That programs of weight control and studies of obesity development during the growing years should begin before the high school period was confirmed by our finding that most of the students who were obese in the twelfth grade were already obese when they were in the ninth grade. Only about two percent of the subjects became obese during this period in their lives. The implied early development of obesity is in line with the findings of others as pointed out in a review by Mossberg (1948) and confirmed in the recent retrospective study of Heald and Hollander (1965).

We noted differences in body height between lean and obese youngsters. Obese boys were taller than other boys especially in the ninth grade. Perhaps this was an indication that the fast-growing, early-maturing boy was more inclined to obesity. However, the opposite was true for girls. In all grades, the lean and somewhat lean girls were taller than other girls. This greater height for the leaner girls did not seem to indicate greater maturity, because we found, in comparing ages at which menstruation began, that the obese girls did mature earlier than the lean girls. For both boys and girls, the gain in stature from ninth to twelfth grades was greater for the lean subjects than for the obese. Perhaps more study should be done in this area before we draw conclusions. However, these findings suggest that tall boys and short girls may be more likely to develop obesity and therefore should be more carefully observed for this tendency.

One of the changes we saw in the entire sample during the high school years was that both boys and girls were still growing, the boys more rapidly. In boys the significant, though not large, increase in body fat occurred from the eleventh to the twelfth grade when their increase in height was the least. The girls increased in body fat from the tenth to the eleventh grade and decreased again by the twelfth grade. We thought the earlier increase might reflect normal development, and the later decrease might be caused by voluntary weight reduction. (The girls' questionnaire responses indicated a growing concern in this area.) To us this growth meant that teenagers do indeed need good diets. Teenage girls, if they are going to restrict their calories, particularly need guidance to select nutritious, low-calorie diets.

We found differences in many measurements which indicated to us that the same standards for size and growth should not be applied to all races. Negro boys and girls have smaller bi-iliac and bitrochanteric diameters in relation to their height than do Oriental or Caucasian boys and girls. Oriental and Negro teenagers both have larger biacromial diameters than do Caucasians when this measurement is related to height. Oriental boys and girls tend to have generally larger diameters for their height than others. Because of these differences in skeletal proportion, we separated the ethnic groups when comparing anthropometric values that might characterize the lean or obese. We found that within each racial group the bitrochanteric diameter particularly was larger for height in obese teenagers. Although obese boys and girls tend to have broader bone structure in relation to heights than do other groups, the predictive value of broad bone structure in anticipating future obesity seems to be fairly good for boys and poor for girls. (This last observation is based on the very small number of subjects who became obese while we were studying them. It included only six boys and twelve girls.) We hope that more definitive work can be done in this area of identifying individuals who may become obese because we feel that it would be helpful to clinicians to be able to estimate the potential of a patient to become obese or remain lean.

A larger proportion of the Negro boys and girls were classified as obese and somewhat obese than Caucasian boys or girls. A much smaller percentage of Oriental boys and girls were classified this way. Does this mean that Negro children are particularly vulnerable to obesity development and, therefore, should be carefully watched to ward off obesity at its onset?

Regardless of which method of classification we used for dividing our subjects into socioeconomic groups, we found teenagers in the lower socioeconomic group to be fatter than others. The lower groups, however, were composed of a disproportionate number of Negroes. Orientals, also, tended to fall in the lower socioeconomic groups. Negroes had more and Orientals less tendency toward obesity than the Caucasians.

Attitudes

The popular impression that teenagers are keenly interested in the size and shape of their developing figures was well documented by our study. The predominant attitude that these students expressed was dissatisfaction—with their weight, fatness or leanness, height, and certain other body dimensions.

More than half the girls expressed concern about overweight, about matching the number of boys who were concerned about being underweight. Boys generally wanted to be taller, while girls seemed to be content with their height. Nearly all the boys expressed a desire for larger biceps, and almost all the girls wanted smaller waists.

The number of girls who described themselves as too fat increased from 43 percent in the ninth grade to 56 percent in the twelfth grade. And some who did not feel they were too fat still wanted to lose weight because 70 percent of the girls desired a weight loss. Less than one-fourth of the boys felt they were too fat. We think this interest and concern can be used effectively to provide channels to reach teenagers with good nutritional information. Certainly they demonstrated a need for more information in the answers to a question about the foods needed daily for health. When replies to this question were evaluated using the "Basic Four" (U.S.D.A., 1958) food groups, fruits and vegetables, and also meat were mentioned more frequently than milk by both boys and girls. Cereal grain foods were not commonly considered essential. Frequent mention of items such as sugar, fats, and vitamin supplements suggested that a number of students may have been somewhat confused by what they had heard from one source or another. About half the subjects failed to mention all four of the basic food groups. This seems a fairly good indication that the work of the nutrition educator is not yet done.

Activity

Our girls averaged more than 95 percent of their time in sleeping, very light, and light activity; our boys averaged more than 90 percent of their time in these categories. Both boys and girls spent on the average nearly 80 percent of their time in either sitting or lying down (sleep and very light activity, an energy expenditure of less than 2.5 calories per minute). It is clear that these teenagers were a remarkably inactive group. There is no reason to expect these inactive teenagers to become more active physically as they grow into adulthood. This raises some questions of importance to health workers. Has the time come when we really should emphasize increased physical activity? If so, how can people be motivated to spend their leisure time in more active ways?

We found poor correlation between low levels of activity and larger amounts of body fat. The gross measurement of physical activity that we used is probably inadequate to distinguish individual differences in levels of total energy expenditure. However, it does serve to identify general patterns of activity.

Eating Practices

What and how did these teenagers eat? Our subjects did not eat very much. The girls managed to get along on less than 2,000 calories a day although the Recommended Allowance is 2,300 calories, while the boys consumed about 2,850 calories a day, quite a bit below the Recommended Allowances of the National Research Council of 3,400 calories a day. In spite of this the boys got an average of all nutrients very close to Recommended Allowances. The girls, as might be expected from their fairly low caloric intakes, had mean values for some nutrients below Recommended Allowances. The average intake of iron of all girls was below two-thirds of the Recommended Allowances, and their mean intake of calcium was only slightly above this level. On the other hand, the girls' mean intakes for vitamins were all at or above the Recommended Allowance level (Food and Nutrition Board, 1964). (From here on the unqualified term "low intake" will indicate below two-thirds of the Recommended Daily Allowances.) Nearly 20 percent of the boys had low intakes of calcium, and 30 percent had intakes low in ascorbic acid, even though the average intake of ascorbic acid was well above Recommended Allowances. Fifty percent of the girls had low intakes of calcium and 60 percent had low levels of iron in their diets. Do we need to suggest iron supplementation for this age group? Fifteen percent had low intakes of vitamin A and ascorbic acid. Among boys and girls with low calcium intakes, there was a general tendency to substitute soft drinks for milk at mealtime.

What differences in diet can we find among youngsters in different body fat categories? The average boys tended to have higher caloric intakes than lean or obese boys. The lean girls tended to have a higher intake of calories than average or obese girls. In general, a higher caloric intake was associated with a higher intake of protein, minerals, and vitamins. Obese and somewhat obese teenagers tended to have poorer diets than others. There was a tendency for obese boys and girls to snack less frequently than other boys and girls, and also a tendency for the obese teenagers to skip meals more often than other teenagers.

Negro teenagers and those in the lower socioeconomic groups tended to have lower intakes of food nutrients than other boys and girls. We have noted that teenagers in these categories are more likely to be obese. These findings suggest a need for more nutrition education and perhaps food or income supplementation for these groups.

We found that teenagers tended to omit meals and snack often. In addition, roughly one-third of the subjects and, in particular, 90 percent of the Negro teenagers had highly irregular eating practices that suggest a way of living and eating quite different from the traditional three-meal-a-day pattern. It was apparent that many youngsters were fending for themselves. Some were buying their own snacks and meals away from home while others were apparently helping themselves to whatever they could find in refrigerator or cupboard. Ethnic classification appeared more closely associated with eating patterns than socioeconomic grouping in that Negroes had less regular patterns. In general, those teenagers who ate regular structured meals, usually augmented by snacks, tended to have better diets than the irregular eaters. Obviously, a change to regular meal eating would necessitate a change in the entire way of life for the irregular eaters and for their families as well. Is this a realistic goal for nutrition educators? Should home economics and nutrition teaching change its emphasis from meal-planning to buying of nutritious snacks and convenience foods that can serve as snacks? It was apparent that if these children were to have nutritious food, it had to be readily available to them. Certainly we can depend on teenagers to eat snacks.

ASSOCIATION FOR ACTIVITY AND EATING PRACTICES WITH OBESITY. As indicated previously, we found poor correlation between body fatness and levels of activity and also between fatness and caloric intake. Our measurements of both activity and food intake were admittedly gross, such as one might reasonably employ with a free-living population. In order to reconcile our findings with the law of the conservation of energy, i.e. that caloric intake must balance caloric storage and expenditure, we must conclude that apparent discrepancies lie in the area of (1) basal energy requirements (not measured in our subjects), (2) efficiency in energy absorption and utilization (probably genetically determined), or (3) those differences in overt activity and food intake not measured by our tools. It is our opinion that differences in basal requirements and seemingly small differences in activity and food intake, perhaps combined with genetically determined differences in efficiency of energy utilization, are indeed adequate to account for varying degrees of fatness. Total average energy intakes and presumably the energy needs of our subjects were not high. We recognize that basal needs might vary by several hundred calories per day and still fall within the generally accepted normal range of ±20 percent of mean. Overt activity might also vary by this much or more without being readily observable. Small additive differences in quantity, or composition of food likewise easily amount to the energy value of a pound of human flesh. It is therefore not necessary to invoke the specters of either laziness or gluttony to account for obesity when energy requirements in general are low. By the same token, small adjustments in food intake and activity can make the difference, over time, between "normal" body composition and obesity. Recognition of this fact should be encouraging to all who are interested in obesity prevention.

RECENT CHANGES. Since the collection of the data reported in this study, changes in life-style have occurred among Berkeley teenagers. The "counter-culture" movement with its emphasis on vegetarianism and use of "organic" and "natural" foods has made its impact. We have no information regarding the number or percentage of young people who may have changed to vegetarianism or other forms of dietary restriction. Nor do we know as a result of this movement its effect on nutrient intakes. These matters need to be investigated. With the movement has come an interest in nutrition that should be exploited for sound, nutritional education.

BIBLIOGRAPHY

The American and his diet. *Lancet, 1*:1373, 1964.

Beaudoin, R., and Mayer, J.: Food intakes of obese and nonobese women. *J AM Diet Assoc, 29*:29, 1953.

Behnke, A. R.: Anthropometric estimate of body size, shape, and fat content. *Postgrad Med, 34*:190, 1963a.

Behnke, A. R.: Anthropometric evaluation of body composition throughout life. *Ann NY Acad Sci, 110*:450, Part II, 1963b.

Behnke, A. R.: Quantitative assessment of body build. *J Appl Physiol, 16*:960, 1961.

Behnke, A. R. and Wilmore, J. T.: *Evaluation and Regulation of Body Build and Composition.* New York, Acad Pr, 1972.

Behnke, A. R., Feen, B. G., and Welham, W. C.: The specific gravity of health men. *JAMA, 118*:495, 1942.

Bullen, B. A., Monello, L. F., Cohen, H., and Mayer, J.: Attitudes towards physical activity, food, and family in obese and nonobese adolescent girls. *Am J Clin Nutr, 12*:1, 1963.

California State Department of Education, Bureau of Health Education, Physical Education and Recreation: *The Physical Performance Test for California, 1966.* Sacramento, California Office of State Printing, 1966.

Deischer, R. W., and Mills, C. A.: The adolescent looks at his health and medical care. *Am J Public Health, 53*:1928, 1963.

Eppright, E. S., Sidwell, V. D., and Jebe, E.: Food intake and body size of Iowa children. *Weight Control* (a collection of papers presented at the Weight Control Colloquium). Ames, The Iowa State College Press, 1955, pp. 119–331.

Eppright, E. S., Sidwell, V. D., and Swanson, P. P.: Nutritive value of the diets of Iowa children. *J Nutr, 54*:371, 1954.

Falkner, F.: Skeletal maturation; an appraisal of concept and method. *Am J Phys Anthropol, 16*:381, 1958.

Food and Agriculture Organization of the United Nations: *Calorie Requirements.* Rome, Nutritional Studies No. 15, 1957.

Food and Nutrition Board: Recommended dietary allowances. Washington, D.C., publication no. 1146, National Academy of Science, National Research Council, 1964.

Forbes, G. B.: Growth of the lean body mass during childhood and adolescence. *J Pediatr, 64:*822, 1964.

Forbes, G. B., Gallup, J. and Hursh, J. B.: 1961. Estimation of total body fat from potassium 40 content. *Science, 133:*101, 1961.

Garn, S. M., and Haskell, J. A.: Fat and growth during childhood. *Science, 130:*1711, 1959.

Guttman, L.: A basis for scaling qualitative data. *Am Sociol Rev, 9:*139, 1944.

Hampton, M. C., Shapiro, L. R., and Huenemann, R. L.: Helping teenage girls improve their diets. *J Home Econ, 53:*835, 1961.

Heald, F. P., Daugela, M., and Brunschuyler, P.: Physiology of adolescence. *N Engl J Med, 268:*243, 1963.

Heald, F., and Hollander, R.: The relationship between obesity in adolescence and early growth". *J Pediatr, 67:*35, 1965.

Hinkle, E. L., Plummer, N., Metraux, R., Richter, P., Gittinger, J. W., Thetford, W. N., Ostfeld, A. M., Kane, F. D., Goldberger, L., Mitchell, W. E., Leichter, H., Pinsky, R., Goebel, D., Bross, I. D. J., and Wolff, H. G.: Studies in human ecology, factors relevant to the occurrence of bodily illness and disturbances in mood, thought and behavior in three homogeneous population groups. *Am J Psychiatry, 114:*212, 1957.

Hinton, M. A.: Factors related to the eating behavior and dietary adequacy of girls 12 to 14 years of age. Ph.D. dissertation, Iowa State University of Science and Technology, 1962.

Hinton, M. A., Eppright, E. S., Chadderdon, H., and Wolins, L.: Eating behavior and dietary intake of girls 12 to 14 years old. *J Am Diet Assoc, 43:*223, 1963.

Hodges, R. E., and Krehl, W. A.: Nutritional status of teen-agers in Iowa. *Am J Clin Nutr, 17:*200, 1965.

Hollingshead, A. B.: *Two Factor Index of Social Position.* New Haven, 1965 Yale Station, 1957.

Hollingshead, A. B., and Redlich, F. C.: *Social Class and Mental Illness: a Community Study.* New York, Wiley, 1958 (Appendix 2).

Horwitt, M. K.: Niacin-tryptophan requirements of man. *J Am Diet Assoc, 34:*914, 1958.

Huenemann, R. L., Hampton, M. C., Shapiro, L. R., and Behnke, A. R.: Adolescent food practices associated with obesity. *Fed Proc, 25:*4, 1966.

Hutson, E. M., Cohen, N. L., Kunkel, N. D., Steinkamp, R. C., Rourke, M. H., and Walsh, H. E.: Measures of body fat and related factors in normal adults. III. Diet and physical activity. *J Am Diet Assoc, 47:*179, 1965.

Iowa Child Welfare Research Station: *Paper Scale for Measuring Children and Adults in English and Metric Units.* Iowa City, University of Iowa, 1925.

Jalso, S. B., Burns, M. M., and Rivers, J. M.: Nutritional beliefs and practices. *J Am Diet Assoc, 47:*263, 1965.

Johnson, M. L., Burke, B. S., and Mayer, J.: Relative importance of inactivity and overeating in the energy balance of obese high school girls. *Am J Clin Nutr, 4:*37, 1956.

Jones, H. E.: 1938. The California adolescent growth study. *J Educ Research, 31:*561, 1938.

Keys, A., and Brozek, J.: Body fat in adult man. *Physiol Rev, 33:*245, 1953.

Litman, T. J., Cooney, J. P., and Stief, R.: The views of Minnesota school children on food. *J Am Diet Assoc, 45:*433, 1964.

Mann, G. V., Shaffer, R. D., Anderson, R. S., and Sandstead, H. H.: Cardiovascular disease in the Masai. *J Atheroscler Res, 4:*289, 1964.

Metropolitan Life Insurance Co.: New Weight Standards for Men and Women. *Stat Bull Metropol Life Ins Co, 40:*1, November–December, 1959.

Morgan, A. F. (Ed.): Nutritional status U.S.A. *California Agric Exper Sta Bull No. 769,* 1959.

Mossberg, H. O.: Obesity in children; clinical-prognostical investigation. *Acta Paediatr, 35:*1, Suppl. 2, 1948.

Murphy, G. E., Robins, E., Kuhn, N. O., and Christensen, R. F.: Stress, sickness and psychiatric disorder in a 'normal' population: A study of 101 young women. *J Nerv Ment Dis, 134:*228, 1962.

Passmore, R., and Durnin, J. V. G. A.: Human energy expenditure. *Physiol Rev, 35:*801, 1955.

Pryor, H. B.: Certain physical and physiological aspects of adolescent development in girls. *J Pediatr, 8:*52, 1936.

Reynolds, E. L.: Sexual maturation and growth of fat, muscle, and bone in girls. *Child Dev, 17:*121, 1946.

Scheffe, H.: On solutions of the Behrens-Fisher problem based on the 't' distribution. *Ann Math Stat, 14:*35, 1943.

Seltzer, C. C., and Mayer, J.: Body build and obesity—who are the obese? *JAMA, 189:*677, 1964.

Siri, W. E.: The gross composition of the body. *Advances in Biological and Medical Physics, 4:*239, 1956.

Stefanik, P. A., Heald, F. P., and Mayer, J.: Caloric intake in relation to energy output of obese and non-obese adolescent boys. *Am J Clin Nutr, 7:*55, 1959.

Stuart, H. C.: Physical growth during adolescence, *Am J Dis Child, 74:*495, 1947.

Stunkard, A. J., Grace, W. J., and Wolff, H. G.: The night-eating syndrome: A pattern of food intake among certain obese patients. *Am J Med, 19:*78, 1955.

Tanner, J. M.: *Growth at Adolescence.* Springfield, Thomas, 1955.

Tanner, J. M.: *Growth at Adolescence,* 2nd ed. Oxford, Blackwell Scientific Publications, 1966, 3rd printing.

Tanner, J. M.: *The Physique of the Olympic Athlete.* London, George Allen and Unwin Ltd., 1964.

The American and his diet. *Lancet, 1*:1373, 1964.

Trulson, M. F., Clancy, R. E., Jessop, W. J. E., Childers, R. W., and Stare, F. J.: Comparisons of siblings in Boston and Ireland. *J Am Diet Assoc, 45*:225, 1964.

Tuddenham, R. D., Snyder, M. M.: Physical growth of California boys and girls from birth to eighteen years. *University of California Publication in Child Development*, vol. 1, no. 2. Berkeley and Los Angeles, U of Cal Pr, 1954.

U.S. Census of Population: Income in 1959 of families and persons, and weeks worked in 1959 for standard metropolitan statistical areas, urbanized areas, and urban places of 10,000 and more. California, General Social and Economic Characteristics, Final Report PC910–6D, 1960, Table 76.

U.S.D.A.: *Food for Fitness: A Daily Food Guide.* leaflet no. 424, 1958.

U.S. Department of Health, Education and Welfare; Heart disease Control Program, Division of Chronic Diseases, Public Health Service: *Dietary Appraisal Using the IBM 7090 Computer.* Mimeo. bulletin, Washington, D.C., 1964

Washburn, A. H.: The child as a person developing. I. A philosophy and program of research. *Am J Dis Child, 94*:46, 1957.

Wetzel, N. C.: Physical fitness in terms of physique, development and basal metabolism. *JAMA, 116*:1187, 1941.

Withers, R. F. J.: Problems in the genetics of human obesity. *The Eugenics Review 56*:81, no. 2, 1964.

Young, C. M., Berresford, K., and Waldner, B. G.: What the homemaker knows about nutrition. III. Relation of knowledge to practice. *J Am Diet Assoc, 32*:321, 1956.

Young, C. M., Martin, M. E. K., Chihan, M., McCarthy, M., Manniello, M. J., Harmuth, E. H., Fryer, J. H.: Body composition of young women, *J Am Diet Assoc, 38*:332, 1961.

APPENDICES

QUINTILE RANGES OF BODY MEASUREMENTS FOR FOUR YEARS

TABLE I

QUINTILE RANGES NINTH GRADE MEASUREMENTS

All Boys (458) (Age: 14.49) | *All Girls* (519) (Age: 14.51)

Height (dm)

All Boys	n	50th P	All Girls	n	50th P
13.62–15.82	= 92		14.57–15.62(1) *	= 104	
15.84–16.39(1) *	= 91	50th P: 16.625	(1)15.62–15.99(1)	= 104	50th P: 16.17
(2)16.39–16.87	= 92		(2)15.99–16.35(3)	= 103	
16.88–17.38	= 91		(2)16.35–16.71(1)	= 104	
17.40–18.95	= 92		(2)16.71–17.90	= 104	

Weight (kg)

All Boys	n	50th P	All Girls	n	50th P
27.70–46.40	= 92		34.30–47.80(2)	= 104	
46.50–51.80(1)	= 91	50th P: 54.10	(4)47.80–51.90(2)	= 104	50th P: 54.00
(2)51.80–56.50	= 92		(2)51.90–56.00(2)	= 103	
56.80–62.70	= 91		(2)56.00–61.40(1)	= 104	
63.10–129.20	= 92		(2)61.40–94.00	= 104	

Shoulder Circumference (cm)

All Boys	n	50th P	All Girls	n	50th P
75.50–92.50	= 92		80.90–91.80	= 104	
92.60–96.70	= 91	50th P: 98.70	91.90–95.00(5)	= 104	50th P: 96.20
96.80–100.50(2)	= 92		(2)95.00–97.40(4)	= 103	
(1)100.50–105.20	= 91		(1)97.40–100.50	= 104	
105.30–135.30	= 92		100.60–127.20	= 104	

Chest Circumference (cm)

All Boys	n	50th P	All Girls	n	50th P
62.40–75.70(3)	= 92		68.20–78.50(3)	= 104	
(1)75.70–79.30	= 91	50th P: 81.50	(3)78.50–81.20(3)	= 104	50th P: 82.50
79.50–83.50(2)	= 92		(5)81.20–83.50(7)	= 103	
(6)83.50–87.00(2)	= 91		(1)83.50–86.30(1)	= 104	
(3)87.00–120.20	= 92		(1)86.30–105.80	= 104	

Upper Abdomen Circumference (cm)

All Boys	n	50th P	All Girls	n	50th P
54.80–63.30(1)	= 92		54.60–61.70	= 104	
(1)63.30–66.20(4)	= 91	50th P: 67.30	61.80–64.10(2)	= 104	50th P: 65.30
(5)66.20–68.50(8)	= 92		(1)64.10–66.40	= 103	
(1)68.50–72.50(1)	= 91		66.50–69.60	= 104	
(2)72.50–108.10	= 92		69.70–107.30	= 104	

Lower Abdomen Circumference (cm)

All Boys	n	50th P	All Girls	n	50th P
54.50–65.10(1)	= 92		60.80–71.20(1)	= 104	
(3)65.10–67.80(1)	= 91	50th P: 68.80	(3)71.20–74.60(2)	= 104	50th P: 75.90
(3)67.80–70.30(4)	= 92		(1)74.60–77.30	= 103	
(3)70.30–74.80	= 91		77.40–81.80	= 104	
75.00–119.00	= 92		81.90–119.00	= 104	

Buttocks Circumference (cm)

All Boys	n	50th P	All Girls	n	50th P
63.80–78.40(1)	= 92		72.30–86.80(2)	= 104	
(2)78.40–81.80	= 91	50th P: 83.30	(1)86.80–90.60(4)	= 104	50th P: 92.00
81.90–84.70(2)	= 92		(1)90.60–93.50(4)	= 103	
(1)84.70–89.40(2)	= 91		(1)93.50–97.20(2)	= 104	
(1)89.40–124.50	= 92		(1)97.20–121.60	= 104	

Lean Body Weight (kg)

All Boys	n	50th P	All Girls	n	50th P
24.93–42.02	= 92		31.76–40.53	= 104	
42.10–46.18(2)	= 91	50th P: 48.805(NC) **	40.54–43.99(1)	= 104	50th P: 45.09(NC) **
(1)46.18–50.53	= 92		(1)43.99–46.01(2)	= 103	
50.63–55.51	= 91		(1)46.01–49.74	= 104	
55.53–78.35	= 92		49.76–63.07	= 104	

Average Calf Circumference (cm)

All Boys	n	50th P	All Girls	n	50th P
26.15–31.04	= 92		26.91–32.00(2)	= 104	
31.10–32.36	= 91	50th P: 33.01	(4)32.00–33.35(10)	= 104	50th P: 33.90
32.42–33.73(1)	= 92		(2)33.35–34.63(5)	= 103	
(1)33.73–35.46	= 91		(2)34.63–36.17	= 104	
35.52–49.75	= 92		36.23–44.07	= 104	

Average Ankle Circumference (cm)

All Boys	n	50th P	All Girls	n	50th P
16.74–20.20(4)	= 92		17.50–20.02	= 104	
(2)20.20–20.92(1)	= 91	50th P: 21.38	20.09–20.79(1)	= 104	50th P: 21.13
(3)20.92–21.78(4)	= 92		(5)20.79–21.53(2)	= 103	
(3)21.78–22.72(1)	= 91		(7)21.53–22.39(3)	= 104	
(2)22.72–30.13	= 92		(5)22.39–26.38	= 104	

Average Abdomen Circumference (cm)

All Boys	n	50th P	All Girls	n	50th P
55.00–64.10(2)	= 92		58.90–66.50	= 104	
(2)64.10–66.85	= 91	50th P: 68.025(NC)	66.55–69.30	= 104	50th P: 70.55
66.90–69.40(4)	= 92		69.35–71.80	= 103	
(2)69.40–73.50	= 91		71.85–75.60(1)	= 104	
73.60–113.55	= 92		75.60–110.40	= 104	

* Number in parentheses means number of students in the range with that particular measurement.
** NC = No child with this particular measurement.

TABLE I (Cont'd.)

All Boys (458) (Age: 14.49)	n		All Girls (519) (Age: 14.51)	n	

Average Biceps Circumference (cm)

All Boys (458) (Age: 14.49)	n		All Girls (519) (Age: 14.51)	n	
19.70–24.35	= 92		19.75–24.25	= 104	
24.40–25.90(4)	= 91	50th P: 26.70	24.30–25.35(3)	= 104	50th P: 25.90
(1)25.90–27.60(1)	= 92		(3)25.35–26.40(4)	= 103	
(3)27.60–29.10(1)	= 91		(1)26.40–27.85	= 104	
(1)29.10–39.50	= 92		27.90–37.05	= 104	

Average Forearm Circumference (cm)

All Boys	n		All Girls	n	
18.65–22.25	= 92		18.50–21.65	= 104	
22.30–23.40(5)	= 91	50th P: 23.90	21.70–22.60(8)	= 104	50th P: 23.75
(2)23.40–24.45	= 92		(1)22.60–23.30(4)	= 103	
24.50–25.45(4)	= 91		(4)23.30–24.20(3)	= 104	
(2)25.45–31.85	= 92		(2)24.20–29.00	= 104	

Average Wrist Circumference (cm)

All Boys	n		All Girls	n	
12.80–15.00(8)	= 92		13.10–14.60(11)	= 104	
(1)15.00–15.55(3)	= 91	50th P: 15.80	(7)14.60–15.00(9)	= 104	50th P: 15.20
(4)15.55–16.00(8)	= 92		(6)15.00–15.45(2)	= 103	
(2)16.00–16.65(1)	= 91		(10)15.45–15.75(16)	= 104	
(7)16.65–18.80	= 92		(2)15.75–18.10	= 104	

Average Knee Circumference (cm)

All Boys	n		All Girls	n	
26.80–32.60	= 92		29.30–33.00	= 104	
32.65–33.70(2)	= 91	50th P: 34.15	33.05–34.30(5)	= 104	50th P: 34.80
(8)33.70–34.65(1)	= 92		(3)34.30–35.40(4)	= 103	
(4)34.65–36.10(7)	= 91		(3)35.40–36.75(1)	= 104	
(1)36.10–50.35	= 92		(2)36.75–44.95	= 104	

Average Thigh Circumference (kg)

All Boys	n		All Girls	n	
35.80–45.55(1)	= 92		41.20–52.30	= 104	
(1)45.55–47.85(2)	= 91	50th P: 49.00	52.35–54.80(1)	= 104	50th P: 56.30
(5)47.85–50.30(1)	= 92		(2)54.80–57.50	= 103	
(1)50.30–53.85(1)	= 91		57.60–60.95	= 104	
(1)53.85–80.75	= 92		61.05–78.95	= 104	

Chest Diameter (cm)

All Boys	n		All Girls	n	
20.10–24.00(6)	= 92		20.20–23.90(9)	= 104	
(2)24.00–25.00(14)	= 91	50th P: 25.70	(1)23.90–24.80(8)	= 104	50th P: 25.10
(3)25.00–26.20(4)	= 92		(12)24.80–25.50(10)	= 103	
(3)26.20–27.50(4)	= 91		(9)25.50–26.40(7)	= 104	
(2)27.50–37.20	= 92		(5)26.40–31.20	= 104	

Bitrochanteric Diameter (cm)

All Boys	n		All Girls	n	
21.00–27.70(9)	= 92		26.40–29.10(6)	= 104	
(1)27.70–29.00(6)	= 91	50th P: 29.70	(2)29.10–30.30(2)	= 104	50th P: 30.80
(3)29.00–30.20(2)	= 92		(4)30.30–31.20	= 103	
(4)30.20–31.50(7)	= 91		31.30–32.30(6)	= 104	
(1)31.50–39.10	= 92		(3)32.30–39.70	= 104	

Wrist Diameter (cm)

All Boys	n		All Girls	n	
8.50–10.10	= 92		7.90– 9.30(24)	= 104	
10.20–10.50(17)	= 91	50th P: 10.70	(9)9.30– 9.60(19)	= 104	50th P: 9.75(NC) **
(8)10.50–10.90(2)	= 92		(18)9.60– 9.90(13)	= 103	
(18)10.90–11.30(1)	= 91		(25)9.90–10.20(17)	= 104	
(13)11.30–12.30	= 92		(14)10.20–13.70	= 104	

Ankle Diameter (cm)

All Boys	n		All Girls	n	
11.60–13.10(5)	= 92		9.20–11.80(11)	= 104	
(10)13.10–13.70(11)	= 91	50th P: 13.90	(14)11.80–12.10(25)	= 104	50th P: 12.30
(16)13.70–14.00(21)	= 92		(11)12.10–12.40(13)	= 103	
(15)14.00–14.30(19)	= 91		(26)12.40–12.80(9)	= 104	
(1)14.30–15.80	= 92		(24)12.80–14.20	= 104	

Bi-iliac Diameter (cm)

All Boys	n		All Girls	n	
20.00–24.00(1)	= 92		22.10–24.70(2)	= 104	
(10)24.00–25.10(3)	= 91	50th P: 25.50	(3)24.70–25.70(4)	= 104	50th P: 26.10
(6)25.10–26.00(5)	= 92		(6)25.70–26.50(14)	= 103	
(7)26.00–27.10(1)	= 91		(3)26.50–27.50(14)	= 104	
(3)27.10–32.50	= 92		(1)27.50–35.00	= 104	

Biacromial Diameter (cm)

All Boys	n		All Girls	n	
25.00–34.50(2)	= 92		30.10–33.70	= 104	
(6)34.50–35.90(4)	= 91	50th P: 36.60	33.80–34.90(1)	= 104	50th P: 35.20
(1)35.90–37.00(15)	= 92		(12)34.90–35.80(2)	= 103	
(1)37.00–38.80(5)	= 91		(12)35.80–36.70(4)	= 104	
(1)38.80–44.10	= 92		(5)36.70–40.60	= 104	

Per Cent Body Fat

All Boys	n		All Girls	n	
− 8.14–(+)5.38	= 92		− 3.40–(+)10.34	= 104	
+ 5.42– 9.03	= 91	50th P: 10.67	+10.39–14.97	= 104	50th P: 16.56(NC) **
+ 9.11–12.06	= 92		+15.00–18.40	= 103	
+12.16–16.52	= 91		+18.42–23.36	= 104	
+16.61–41.25	= 92		+23.39–39.15	= 104	

TABLE II
QUINTILE RANGES TENTH-GRADE MEASUREMENTS

All Boys (454) (Age: 15.32)		All Girls (452) (Age: 15.24)	

Height (dm)

	n			n	
14.44–16.52(1)*	= 91		14.26–15.72(3)	= 90	
(2)16.52–16.88	= 91	50th P: 17.13	(3)15.72–16.12(3)	= 91	50th P: 16.29(NC)**
16.89–17.35(1)	= 90		(1)16.12–16.50	= 90	
(7)17.35–17.72	= 91		16.52–16.83(1)	= 91	
17.74–19.45	= 91		(5)16.83–17.96	= 90	

Weight (kg)

33.80–52.70(2)	= 91		36.30–49.00(1)	= 90	
(3)52.70–57.60(4)	= 91	50th P: 59.50	(1)49.00–53.20(2)	= 91	50th P: 55.45
(2)57.60–62.30(1)	= 90		(1)53.20–57.40(2)	= 90	
(1)62.30–68.00	= 91		(2)57.40–62.90	= 91	
68.10–127.90	= 91		63.00–102.60	= 90	

Shoulder Circumference (cm)

83.60–97.80(1)	= 91		81.60–94.20(2)	= 90	
(1)97.80–102.00(3)	= 91	50th P: 104.00	(1)94.20–97.10	= 91	50th P: 98.50
(4)102.00–105.70(2)	= 90		97.20–99.60(2)	= 90	
(1)105.70–110.00(3)	= 91		(1)99.60–102.50(1)	= 91	
(2)110.00–135.50	= 91		(1)102.50–129.00	= 90	

Chest Circumference (cm)

65.80–79.30(2)	= 91		71.00–79.90(2)	= 90	
(1)79.30–83.30	= 91	50th P: 85.00	(2)79.90–82.50(7)	= 91	50th P: 83.55(NC) **
83.40–86.80	= 90		(5)82.50–84.60(1)	= 90	
86.90–90.40(2)	= 91		(1)84.60–87.70(1)	= 91	
(1)90.40–117.70	= 91		(4)87.70–113.00	= 90	

Upper Abdomen Circumference (cm)

55.00–65.30(2)	= 91		54.30–61.50	= 90	
(3)65.30–67.70	= 91	50th P: 69.35(NC)	61.60–63.80(1)	= 91	50th P: 64.90
67.80–70.70(3)	= 90		(2)63.80–66.40(1)	= 90	
(6)70.70–74.20(2)	= 91		(2)66.40–69.60	= 91	
(2)74.20–107.00	= 91		69.80–97.70	= 90	

Lower Abdomen Circumference (cm)

55.00–66.70(1)	= 91		62.00–73.10	= 90	
(5)66.70–69.10	= 91	50th P: 70.60	73.20–76.40	= 91	50th P: 78.40
69.20–72.20(3)	= 90		76.50–80.10	= 90	
(5)72.20–76.00(1)	= 91		80.20–84.70(3)	= 91	
(2)76.00–115.80	= 91		(1)84.70–116.20	= 90	

Buttocks Circumference (cm)

66.50–82.20(1)	= 91		71.30–88.20	= 90	
(2)82.20–85.10	= 91	50th P: 86.40	88.30–91.60(1)	= 91	50th P :93.30(NC) **
85.20–88.00(1)	= 90		(1)91.60–94.70(3)	= 90	
(5)88.00–91.30(3)	= 91		(1)94.70–98.60(3)	= 91	
(1)91.30–123.00	= 91		(3)98.60–121.20	= 90	

Lean Body Weight (kg)

31.68–47.14	= 91		32.94–42.16	= 90	
47.20–51.15	= 91	50th P: 52.95	42.18–45.30	= 91	50th P:46.61(NC) **
51.18–54.71	= 90		45.41–47.70	= 90	
54.74–58.96	= 91		47.89–51.21	= 91	
59.01–80.01	= 91		51.25–65.77	= 90	

Average Calf Circumference (cm)

27.10–32.10	= 91		27.35–32.10(2)	= 90	
32.15–33.55	= 91	50th P: 34.10	(1)32.10–33.65(1)	= 91	50th P: 34.20
33.60–34.75(4)	= 90		(3)33.65–34.75	= 90	
(1)34.75–36.45	= 91		34.80–36.20	= 91	
36.50–49.20	= 91		36.25–45.35	= 90	

Average Ankle Circumference (cm)

17.70–20.85(5)	= 91		17.20–20.00	= 90	
(3)20.85–21.50	= 91	50th P: 21.90	20.05–20.65(6)	= 91	50th P: 21.00
21.55–22.35(1)	= 90		(1)20.65–21.30(6)	= 90	
(7)22.35–23.15	= 91		(1)21.30–22.30(1)	= 91	
23.20–29.75	= 91		(4)22.30–25.90	= 90	

Average Abdomen Circumference (cm)

55.00–65.95	= 91		59.20–67.50	= 90	
66.00–68.50(1)	= 91	50th P: 70.00	67.55–70.25	= 91	50th P: 71.60
(5)68.50–71.35	= 90		70.30–73.20	= 90	
71.40–74.85	= 91		73.25–76.75	= 91	
75.15–111.40	= 91		76.80–106.95	= 90	

* Number in parentheses means number of students in the range with that particular measurement.
** NC = No child with this particular measurement.

Table II (Cont'd.)

All Boys (454) (Age: 15.32) **All Girls (452)** (Age: 15.24)

Average Biceps Circumference (cm)

Boys	n		Girls	n	
20.45–26.10(2)	= 91		20.05–24.05	= 90	
(1)26.10–27.70(1)	= 91	50th P: 28.55	24.10–25.25(2)	= 91	50th P: 25.90
(1)27.70–29.20(3)	= 90		(2)25.25–26.60(1)	= 90	
(3)29.20–30.80(2)	= 91		(3)26.60–28.00	= 91	
(1)30.80–39.80	= 91		28.05–37.15	= 90	

Average Forearm Circumference (cm)

Boys	n		Girls	n	
20.15–23.45	= 91		18.25–21.40(4)	= 90	
23.50–24.60(2)	= 91	50th P: 25.05	(1)21.40–22.30(4)	= 91	50th P: 22.65
(4)24.60–25.40(7)	= 90		(4)22.30–22.95(5)	= 90	
(1)25.40–26.50(6)	= 91		(1)22.95–23.95(2)	= 91	
(1)26.50–31.65	= 91		(6)23.95–29.50	= 90	

Average Wrist Circumference (cm)

Boys	n		Girls	n	
13.85–15.45(7)	= 91		12.60–14.35(10)	= 90	
(2)15.45–16.00(6)	= 91	50th P: 16.15	(3)14.35–14.85(6)	= 91	50th P: 15.05
(11)16.00–16.30(15)	= 90		(3)14.85–15.25(9)	= 90	
(1)16.30–16.85(2)	= 91		(1)15.25–15.70(5)	= 91	
(3)16.85–18.95	= 91		(6)15.70–18.25	= 90	

Average Knee Circumference (cm)

Boys	n		Girls	n	
29.80–33.45(1)	= 91		29.30–34.15(2)	= 90	
(1)33.45–34.50	= 91	50th P: 34.95	(1)34.15–35.35(3)	= 91	50th P: 36.00
34.55–35.40(6)	= 90		(1)35.35–36.55(1)	= 90	
(2)35.40–36.75	= 91		(2)36.55–37.85	= 91	
36.75–48.45	= 91		37.90–48.85	= 90	

Average Thigh Circumference (cm)

Boys	n		Girls	n	
38.50–48.10	= 91		46.15–52.90	= 90	
48.15–50.35	= 91	50th P: 51.45	52.95–55.55	= 91	50th P: 56.45
50.40–52.65(4)	= 90		55.60–57.65(2)	= 90	
(1)52.65–55.85	= 91		(3)57.65–60.70(1)	= 91	
55.90–80.15	= 91		(2)60.70–80.20	= 90	

Chest Diameter (cm)

Boys	n		Girls	n	
22.20–25.00(12)	= 91		21.40–24.00(6)	= 90	
(1)25.00–26.10	= 91	50th P: 26.70	(1)24.00–25.00(4)	= 91	50th P: 25.40
26.20–27.30(3)	= 90		(6)25.00–25.80(4)	= 90	
(8)27.30–28.30	= 91		(8)25.80–26.60(4)	= 91	
28.40–33.10	= 91		(3)26.60–30.80	= 90	

Bitrochanteric Diameter (cm)

Boys	n		Girls	n	
23.60–29.10(7)	= 91		25.80–29.40(9)	= 90	
(2)29.10–30.30(4)	= 91	50th P: 30.80	(1)29.40–30.40(8)	= 91	50th P: 30.9
(4)30.30–31.10(6)	= 90		(1)30.40–31.30(7)	= 90	
(3)31.10–32.30	= 91		(3)31.30–32.40(4)	= 91	
32.40–38.70	= 91		(2)32.40–37.20	= 90	

Wrist Diameter (cm)

Boys	n		Girls	n	
9.10–10.60(3)	= 91		8.10– 9.50(14)	= 90	
(23)10.60–10.90(17)	= 91	50th P: 11.00	(17) 9.50– 9.90(7)	= 91	50th P: 10.00
(20)10.90–11.20(10)	= 90		(15) 9.90–10.10(36)	= 90	
(8)11.20–11.60(31)	= 91		(5)10.10–10.40(23)	= 91	
(22)11.60–13.30	= 91		(6)10.40–11.70	= 90	

Ankle Diameter (cm)

Boys	n		Girls	n	
12.00–13.60(13)	= 91		10.40–11.90(1)	= 90	
(4)13.60–14.00(27)	= 91	50th P: 14.20	(18)11.90–12.20(10)	= 91	50th P: 12.30
(17)14.00–14.40(6)	= 90		(20)12.20–12.40(29)	= 90	
(28)14.40–14.70(17)	= 91		(10)12.40–12.70(26)	= 91	
(2)14.70–16.00	= 91		(6)12.70–14.10	= 90	

Bi-iliac Diameter (cm)

Boys	n		Girls	n	
20.70–24.90(3)	= 91		22.00–25.20(6)	= 90	
(5)24.90–26.00(3)	= 91	50th P: 26.50	(1)25.20–26.20	= 90	50th P: 26.70
(10)26.00–26.90(14)	= 90		26.30–27.20(7)	= 90	
(1)26.90–28.00(6)	= 91		(2)27.20–28.30(5)	= 91	
(1)28.00–34.30	= 91		(5)28.30–34.50	= 90	

Biacromial Diameter (cm)

Boys	n		Girls	n	
30.30–36.00(2)	= 91		30.70–34.30(1)	= 90	
(7)36.00–37.40(1)	= 91	50th P: 37.70	(2)34.30–35.20	= 91	50th P: 35.7
(1)37.40–38.30	= 90		35.30–36.30(10)	= 90	
38.40–39.90	= 91		(2)36.30–37.50(2)	= 91	
40.00–44.50	= 91		(7)37.50–41.20	= 90	

Per Cent Body Fat

Boys	n		Girls	n	
− 9.55–(+)6.17	= 91		− 9.44–(+)10.38	= 90	
+ 6.18– 9.96	= 91	50th P: 11.82(NC) **	+10.43–14.53(1)	= 91	50th P:16.39(NC) **
+10.03–13.30(1)	= 90		(1) +14.53–17.80	= 90	
(1) +13.30–17.49	= 91		+17.82–22.74	= 91	
+17.62–44.56	= 91		+22.84–41.67	= 90	

TABLE III
QUINTILE RANGES ELEVENTH-GRADE MEASUREMENTS

All Boys (466) (Age: 16.36)			All Girls (423) (Age: 16.23)	

	n	*Height* (dm)		n
15.04–16.86(3)	= 93		14.32–15.83(1)	= 85
(3)16.86–17.26	= 93	50th P: 17.44	(2)15.83–16.19(1)	= 85
17.27–17.64(1)	= 94		(3)16.19–16.55	= 84
(4)17.64–18.05(1)	= 93		16.56–16.87(4)	= 85
(1)18.05–19.70	= 93		(2)16.87–18.05	= 85

50th P: 16.33

	n	*Weight* (kg)		n
39.00–57.00(1)	= 93		36.20–49.90	= 85
(1)57.00–61.20(2)	= 93	50th P: 63.60	50.00–54.20(1)	= 85
(1)61.20–65.50	= 94		(4)54.20–57.70	= 84
65.60–71.90	= 93		57.80–62.80(1)	= 85
72.00–134.70	= 93		(1)62.80–106.20	= 85

50th P: 55.85– (NC) **

	n	*Shoulder Circumference* (cm)		n
86.80–101.40	= 93		84.20–93.30	= 85
101.50–105.60	= 93	50th P: 107.20	93.40–96.30(1)	= 85
105.70–108.20(5)	= 94		(3)96.30–99.00(7)	= 84
(3)108.20–112.20(2)	= 93		(1)99.00–102.30(1)	= 85
(1)112.20–139.80	= 93		(2)102.30–130.20	= 85

50th P: 97.50

	n	*Chest Circumference* (cm)		n
69.80–82.80	= 93		70.70–79.50(2)	= 85
82.90–86.20(3)	= 93	50th P: 87.40	(3)79.50–82.00(1)	= 85
(1)86.20–89.20	= 94		82.00–84.30(2)	= 84
89.30–92.50(2)	= 93		(5)84.30–86.90	= 85
(1)92.50–119.00	= 93		87.00–109.80	= 85

50th P: 83.05– (NC) **

	n	*Upper Abdomen Circumference* (cm)		n
58.50–60.60	= 93		53.60–60.60	= 85
66.70–69.50(1)	= 93	50th P: 70.80	60.70–63.10(3)	= 85
(3)69.50–72.20(1)	= 94		(4)63.10–65.00(4)	= 84
(6)72.20–75.20(4)	= 93		(4)65.00–68.40(1)	= 85
(1)75.20–113.40	= 93		(1)68.40–101.20	= 85

50th P: 64.10

	n	*Lower Abdomen Circumference* (cm)		n
58.30–67.70(1)	= 93		56.70–68.60	= 85
(5)67.70–70.90	= 93	50th P: 72.20	68.70–72.20(2)	= 85
71.00–73.40	= 94		(3)72.20–75.40(2)	= 84
73.50–77.50	= 93		(3)75.40–79.00	= 85
77.60–123.50	= 93		79.10–111.40	= 85

50th P: 73.80

	n	*Buttocks Circumference* (cm)		n
72.20–84.00(2)	= 93		79.50–88.50	= 85
(2)84.00–86.80(2)	= 93	50th P: 87.70	88.60–91.60	= 85
(4)86.80–89.30(4)	= 94		91.70–94.50(1)	= 84
(3)89.30–92.30(1)	= 93		(2)94.50–98.00	= 85
(1)92.30–124.20	= 93		98.10–126.40	= 85

50th P: 93.00

	n	*Lean Body Weight* (kg)		n
35.62–50.82(1)	= 93		33.52–41.44	= 85
(1)50.82–54.29	= 93	50th P: 55.93	41.45–44.61	= 85
54.30–57.09(1)	= 94		44.62–47.31(1)	= 84
(1)57.09–61.37	= 93		(1)47.31–50.16	= 85
(1)61.37–83.92	= 93		50.17–62.49	= 85

50th P: 45.96

	n	*Average Calf Circumference* (cm)		n
28.50–32.85(2)	= 93		28.30–32.70(1)	= 85
(1)32.85–34.40(3)	= 93	50th P: 34.90	(1)32.70–33.95(1)	= 85
(1)34.40–35.50(2)	= 94		(5)33.95–35.00(2)	= 84
(1)35.00–37.05	= 93		(1)35.00–36.65(3)	= 85
37.06–49.25	= 93		(1)36.65–45.10	= 85

50th P: 34.45

	n	*Average Ankle Circumference* (cm)		n
17.00–21.00(4)	= 93		17.80–20.15(5)	= 85
(6)21.00–21.70(3)	= 93	50th P: 22.00	(1)20.15–20.85(1)	= 85
(2)21.70–22.45(1)	= 94		(4)20.85–21.55(5)	= 84
(4)22.45–23.40(3)	= 93		(1)21.55–22.40	= 85
(1)23.40–29.85	= 93		22.41–26.35	= 85

50th P: 21.15

	n	*Average Abdomen Circumference* (cm)		n
58.40–67.35(1)	= 93		55.15–64.65	= 85
(2)67.35–70.15	= 93	50th P: 71.50	64.66–67.90(3)	= 85
70.16–72.70	= 94		(1)67.90–70.05(1)	= 84
72.71–76.20(1)	= 93		(3)70.05–73.20	= 85
76.21–118.45	= 93		73.21–106.30	= 85

50th P: 69.00

* Number in parentheses means number of students in the range with that particular measurement.
** NC = No child with this particular measurement.

Table III (Cont'd.)

All Boys (426)
(Age: 16.36)

All Girls (423)
(Age: 16.23)

Average Biceps Circumference (cm)

21.55–27.55(1)	= 93		20.45–24.80(7)	= 85	
(1)27.55–29.05	= 93	50th P: 29.70	(1)24.80–26.00	= 85	50th P: 26.55
29.06–30.25(3)	= 94		26.01–27.05(2)	= 84	
(6)30.25–31.90	= 93		(4)27.05–28.40	= 85	
31.91–40.55	= 93		28.41–40.50	= 85	

Average Forearm Circumference (cm)

21.35–24.35	= 93		18.90–21.75	= 85	
24.36–25.30(5)	= 93	50th P: 25.75	21.76–22.60(4)	= 85	50th P: 22.90
(2)25.31–26.10	= 94		(7)22.60–23.30	= 84	
26.10–27.15(3)	= 93		23.31–24.20	= 85	
(1)27.15–32.05	= 93		24.21–29.65	= 85	

Average Wrist Circumference (cm)

13.80–15.80(4)	= 93		13.30–14.60	= 85	
(6)15.80–16.20(2)	= 93	50th P: 16.35	14.61–15.05	= 85	50th P: 15.30
(8)16.20–16.55(5)	= 94		15.06–15.50(1)	= 84	
(7)16.55–17.05(4)	= 93		(8)15.50–15.85(6)	= 85	
(2)17.05–19.00	= 93		(4)15.85–17.95	= 85	

Average Knee Circumference (cm)

30.10–33.85(2)	= 93		29.10–34.05(4)	= 85	
(4)33.85–34.95(3)	= 93	50th P: 35.30	(2)34.05–35.35(5)	= 85	50th P: 35.95
(4)34.95–35.80(1)	= 94		(3)35.35–36.50	= 84	
(6)35.80–37.00	= 93		36.51–37.95(1)	= 85	
37.01–47.30	= 93		(3)37.95–47.20	= 85	

Average Thigh Circumference (cm)

39.55–49.15	= 93		44.85–53.60(1)	= 85	
49.16–51.35(1)	= 93	50th P: 52.30	(1)53.60–56.10(2)	= 85	50th P: 56.90
(1)51.35–53.40(1)	= 94		(3)56.10–58.00(1)	= 84	
(1)53.40–56.65	= 93		(2)58.00–60.60	= 85	
56.66–82.10	= 93		60.61–82.95	= 85	

Chest Diameter (cm)

21.90–25.80(1)	= 93		20.20–23.20(5)	= 85	
(3)25.80–26.90(9)	= 93	50th P: 27.30	(3)23.20–24.10(2)	= 85	50th P: 24.40
(1)26.90–27.70(8)	= 94		(16)24.10–24.80(4)	= 84	
(1)27.70–29.00(5)	= 93		(2)24.80–25.70(8)	= 85	
(11)28.90–38.80	= 93		(3)25.70–28.30	= 85	

Bitrochanteric Diameter (cm)

25.00–30.00(10)	= 93		25.80–29.50(1)	= 85	
(2)30.00–31.00(14)	= 93	50th P: 31.30	(7)29.50–30.50(10)	= 85	50th P: 30.95
(13)31.00–31.90(4)	= 94		(4)30.50–31.30(1)	= 84	
(7)31.90–33.00(1)	= 93		(7)31.30–32.50(1)	= 85	
(9)33.00–39.60	= 93		(9)32.50–37.70	= 85	

Wrist Diameter (cm)

9.40–10.80(5)	= 93		8.10– 9.20(16)	= 85	
(28)10.80–11.10(11)	= 93	50th P: 11.30	(15) 9.20– 9.50(13)	= 85	50th P: 9.70
(21)11.10–11.40(17)	= 94		(10) 9.50– 9.80(19)	= 84	
(11)11.40–11.80(6)	= 93		(16) 9.80–10.10(14)	= 85	
(12)11.80–13.40	= 93		(12)10.10–11.10	= 85	

Ankle Diameter (cm)

12.20–13.60(7)	= 93		10.20–11.70(7)	= 85	
(11)13.60–14.00(13)	= 93	50th P: 14.20	(14)11.70–12.00(25)	= 85	50th P: 12.20
(23)14.00–14.40(2)	= 94		(5)12.00–12.40(7)	= 84	
(24)14.40–14.80(9)	= 93		(26)12.40–12.70(13)	= 85	
(10)14.80–16.30	= 93		(6)12.70–13.70	= 85	

Bi-iliac Diameter (cm)

21.50–25.40(3)	= 93		22.20–25.30(4)	= 85	
(7)25.40–26.40(5)	= 93	50th P: 26.84	(4)25.30–26.30(6)	= 85	50th P: 26.80
(11)26.40–27.40(5)	= 94		(2)26.30–27.30(1)	= 84	
(5)27.40–28.60(7)	= 93		(6)27.30–28.20(6)	= 85	
(2)28.60–34.90	= 93		(3)28.20–33.20	= 85	

Biacromial Diameter (cm)

31.60–37.10(2)	= 93		31.30–34.50(1)	= 85	
(4)37.10–38.30(7)	= 93	50th P: 38.75	(12)34.50–35.40(7)	= 85	50th P: 35.80
(5)38.30–39.40(7)	= 94		(3)35.40–36.20(6)	= 84	
(4)39.40–40.60(4)	= 93		(11)36.20–37.20(1)	= 85	
(6)40.60–44.60	= 93		(6)37.20–40.80	= 85	

Per Cent Body Fat

− 7.18–(+)6.93	= 93		−11.52–(+)12.50	= 85	
6.94–10.52	= 93	50th P: 12.71	12.51–16.74	= 85	50th P: 18.56
10.53–14.17	= 94		16.75–19.98	= 84	
14.18–17.84	= 93		19.99–24.10	= 85	
17.84–45.49	= 93		24.11–43.50	= 85	

TABLE IV

QUINTILE RANGES TWELFTH-GRADE MEASUREMENTS

All Boys (403) (Age: 17.29) | *All Girls* (404) (Age: 17.23)

Height (dm)

Boys range	n	50th P	Girls range	n	50th P
15.16–17.06(1)	= 80		14.26–15.83	= 80	
(1)17.06–17.51(2)	= 81	50th P: 17.68	15.84–16.20	= 81	50th P: 16.38
(2)17.51–17.85(1)	= 81		16.21–16.61	= 82	
(1)17.85–18.26(2)	= 81		16.62–16.92(5) *	= 81	
(1)18.26–19.66	= 80		(1)16.92–18.14	= 80	

Weight (kg)

43.30–59.50	= 80		36.00–50.20(3)	= 80	
59.60–63.90	= 81	50th P: 65.85(NC) **	(1)50.20–54.50(3)	= 81	50th P: 56.40
64.00–68.40	= 81		(2)54.50–58.70	= 82	
68.50–74.80	= 81		58.80–64.10	= 81	
75.00–141.80	= 80		64.20–110.00	= 80	

Shoulder Circumference (cm)

92.30–104.60	= 80		86.50–94.60	= 80	
104.70–107.10(1)	= 81	50th P: 108.50	94.70–96.90(6)	= 81	50th P: 98.40
(1)107.10–110.20(1)	= 81		(1)96.90–99.50(2)	= 82	
(1)110.20–114.10(1)	= 81		(2)99.50–102.80(5)	= 81	
(1)114.10–144.20	= 80		(1)102.80–135.40	= 80	

Chest Circumference (cm)

74.70–84.20(1)	= 80		73.20–80.20	= 80	
(5)84.20–87.30(3)	= 81	50th P: 88.85(NC) **	80.30–83.00(4)	= 81	50th P: 84.00
(5)87.30–90.20(4)	= 81		(4)83.00–85.10(4)	= 82	
(3)90.20–94.10(1)	= 81		(1)85.10–88.50	= 81	
(2)94.10–126.00	= 80		88.60–114.60	= 80	

Upper Abdomen Circumference (cm)

60.20–68.60	= 80		55.20–62.00	= 80	
68.70–71.00(4)	= 81	50th P: 72.10	62.10–64.60	= 81	50th P: 65.80
(3)71.00–73.20	= 81		64.70–66.90	= 82	
73.30–77.20(2)	= 81		67.00–70.30	= 81	
(1)77.20–118.00	= 80		70.40–104.70	= 80	

Lower Abdomen Circumference (cm)

60.10–69.50(1)	= 80		61.80–73.00(1)	= 80	
(1)69.50–72.00(1)	= 81	50th P: 73.00	(1)73.00–75.80(1)	= 81	50th P: 77.50
(4)72.00–74.70	= 81		(3)75.80–79.00(1)	= 82	
74.80–79.00(2)	= 81		(2)79.00–83.80(3)	= 81	
(2)79.00–128.70	= 80		(1)83.80–126.40	= 80	

Buttocks Circumference (cm)

75.00–85.50	= 80		78.40–89.00	= 80	
85.60–87.90	= 81	50th P: 89.20	89.10–92.10	= 81	50th P: 93.40
88.00–90.30(2)	= 81		92.20–95.20(9)	= 82	
(2)90.30–94.50(1)	= 81		(1)95.20–99.70(3)	= 81	
(1)94.50–130.00	= 80		(1)99.70–128.50	= 80	

Lean Body Weight (kg)

39.63–53.65	= 80		33.87–42.74	= 80	
53.68–56.91	= 81	50th P: 58.232(NC) **	42.77–45.70	= 81	50th P: 47.148–
56.92–59.62	= 81		45.76–48.59	= 82	(NC) **
59.64–64.33	= 81		48.62–52.44	= 81	
64.37–90.08	= 80		52.45–69.41	= 80	

Average Calf Circumference (cm)

29.90–33.15(2)	= 80		28.95–32.70(1)	= 80	
(2)33.15–34.40	= 81	50th P: 35.10	(1)32.70–34.05(4)	= 81	50th P: 34.65
34.45–35.65	= 81		(1)34.05–35.30	= 82	
35.70–37.25(3)	= 81		35.35–36.90(1)	= 81	
(1)37.25–50.70	= 80		(1)36.90–46.25	= 80	

Average Ankle Circumference (cm)

18.80–21.00	= 80		17.55–20.15(6)	= 80	
(2)21.00–21.65(4)	= 81	50th P: 21.95	(1)20.15–20.95(1)	= 81	50th P: 21.20
(6)21.65–22.25(3)	= 81		(4)20.95–21.75(2)	= 82	
(2)22.25–23.30(1)	= 81		(6)21.75–22.50(1)	= 81	
(4)23.30–30.05	= 80		(5)22.50–26.00	= 80	

Average Abdomen Circumference (cm)

60.25–69.35	= 80		59.90–67.50	= 80	
69.40–71.45(1)	= 81	50th P: 72.60	67.60–70.10(1)	= 81	50th P: 71.55
(2)71.45–74.00(1)	= 81		(1)70.10–72.75	= 82	
(1)74.00–78.05	= 81		72.80–76.85	= 81	
78.10–123.35	= 80		77.00–115.55	= 80	

* Number in parentheses means number of students in the range with that particular measurement.
** NC = No child with this particular measurement.

TABLE IV (Cont'd.)

All Boys (403) (Age: 17.29)	n		All Girls (404) (Age: 17.23)	n	
		Average Biceps Circumference (cm)			
22.65–28.25(1)	= 80		21.10–24.60(3)	= 80	
(3)28.25–29.90(2)	= 81	50th P: 30.35	(1)24.60–25.80(2)	= 81	50th P: 26.35
(4)29.90–31.10(2)	= 81		(1)25.80–27.00	= 82	
(2)31.10–32.90(4)	= 81		27.05–28.80	= 81	
(1)32.90–43.25	= 80		28.85–41.95	= 80	
		Average Forearm Circumference (cm)			
21.65–24.95	= 80		19.15–22.20	= 80	
25.00–25.90(2)	= 81	50th P: 26.25	22.25–23.05	= 81	50th P: 23.45
(5)25.90–26.70(1)	= 81		23.10–23.90	= 82	
(1)26.70–27.70(2)	= 81		23.95–24.85(2)	= 81	
(1)27.70–33.25	= 80		(1)24.85–30.15	= 80	
		Average Wrist Circumference (cm)			
14.50–15.90(6)	= 80		13.15–14.60(2)	= 80	
(4)15.90–16.35(1)	= 81	50th P: 16.525(NC) **	(5)14.60–14.95(10)	= 81	50th P: 15.20
(11)16.35–16.75(7)	= 81		(1)14.95–15.40(6)	= 82	
(3)16.75–17.25(4)	= 81		(11)15.40–15.90(3)	= 81	
(3)17.25–18.90	= 80		(10)15.90–18.10	= 80	
		Average Knee Circumference (cm)			
30.65–33.85(4)	= 80		29.40–34.05(1)	= 80	
(1)33.85–34.75(9)	= 81	50th P: 35.275(NC) **	(2)34.05–35.40	= 81	50th P: 36.00
(1)34.75–35.75(3)	= 81		35.45–36.75(2)	= 82	
(1)35.75–37.00(3)	= 81		(3)36.75–38.60(1)	= 81	
(1)37.00–47.00	= 80		(1)38.60–48.30	= 80	
		Average Thigh Circumference (cm)			
40.50–49.65(1)	= 80		42.75–51.95	= 80	
(1)49.65–51.70	= 81	50th P: 52.875(NC) **	52.00–54.50	= 81	50th P: 55.65
51.75–53.80(3)	= 81		54.55–56.85	= 82	
(4)53.80–57.20	= 81		57.00–59.90	= 81	
57.25–82.80	= 80		60.00–78.25	= 80	
		Chest Diameter (cm)			
22.60–26.30(6)	= 80		20.30–23.10(13)	= 80	
(1)26.30–27.40(5)	= 81	50th P: 28.00	(1)23.10–24.20(5)	= 81	50th P: 24.60
(2)27.40–28.40(4)	= 81		(7)24.20–25.00(6)	= 82	
(6)28.40–29.50(6)	= 81		(10)25.00–25.80(6)	= 81	
(4)29.50–33.60	= 80		(6)25.80–29.30	= 80	
		Bitrochanteric Diameter (cm)			
26.20–30.60(3)	= 80		26.30–29.80(4)	= 80	
(2)30.60–31.60(5)	= 81	50th P: 32.00	(2)29.80–30.80(8)	= 81	50th P: 31.20
(7)31.60–32.40(9)	= 81		(6)30.80–31.70	= 82	
(3)32.40–33.60(1)	= 81		31.80–32.90(2)	= 81	
(6)33.60–40.80	= 80		(4)32.90–37.90	= 80	
		Wrist Diameter (cm)			
9.60–10.80(13)	= 80		7.90–9.60(8)	= 80	
(6)10.80–11.20(17)	= 81	50th P: 11.40	(9)9.60–9.90(16)	= 81	50th P: 10.00
(12)11.20–11.50(19)	= 81		(16)9.90–10.20(5)	= 82	
(2)11.50–11.90(4)	= 81		(22)10.20–10.50(13)	= 81	
(15)11.90–13.30	= 80		(4)10.50–11.60	= 80	
		Ankle Diameter (cm)			
12.40–13.70(10)	= 80		10.70–12.10(3)	= 80	
(4)13.70–14.10(17)	= 81	50th P: 14.30	(19)12.10–12.40(15)	= 81	50th P: 12.60
(3)14.10–14.50(9)	= 81		(18)12.40–12.80(1)	= 82	
(24)14.50–14.90(14)	= 81		(32)12.80–13.00(23)	= 81	
(1)14.90–16.60	= 80		(3)13.00–14.40	= 80	
		Bi-iliac Diameter (cm)			
23.10–25.90(2)	= 80		23.10–26.00(2)	= 80	
(9)25.90–26.80(1)	= 81	50th P: 27.20	(8)26.00–27.00(5)	= 81	50th P: 27.50
(4)26.80–27.70(3)	= 81		(1)27.00–28.10(7)	= 82	
(1)27.70–28.80(1)	= 81		(1)28.10–29.30	= 81	
(3)28.80–36.60	= 80		29.40–33.80	= 80	
		Biacromial Diameter (cm)			
32.70–38.20(2)	= 80		31.20–34.30(6)	= 80	
(6)38.20–39.30(6)	= 81	50th P: 39.90	(4)34.30–35.30(2)	= 81	50th P: 35.70
(8)39.30–40.40(9)	= 81		(11)35.30–36.30(6)	= 82	
(6)40.40–41.50(2)	= 81		(3)36.30–37.20(8)	= 81	
(3)41.50–46.00	= 80		(6)37.20–42.00	= 80	
		Per Cent Body Fat			
− 7.23–(+)6.57	= 80		−10.12–(+)10.17	= 80	
+ 6.58–10.18	= 81	50th P: 12.045(NC) **	+10.48–15.03	= 81	50th P: 17.01
+10.24–13.81	= 81		+15.05–18.89	= 82	
+13.85–17.92	= 81		+18.95–23.02	= 81	
+18.09–42.67	= 80		+23.07–43.74	= 80	

MEAN CIRCUMFERENCES, DIAMETERS AND ACCESSORY INFORMATION FOR FOUR YEARS

TABLE V

CIRCUMFERENCES, DIAMETERS AND ACCESSORY INFORMATION FOR ALL BOYS, NINTH GRADE **

	All (458)		Caucasian (267)		Negro (137)		Oriental (44)	
	$\bar{X}$	σ	$\bar{X}$	σ	$\bar{X}$	σ	$\bar{X}$	σ
Circumference (cm)								
Abdomen	69.53	7.636	70.96 *†	7.814	67.69 *	6.539	66.18 †	7.728
Ankle	21.48	1.613	21.80 *†	1.571	21.12 *	1.546	20.57 †	1.583
Biceps	26.96	3.030	27.10	2.972	26.95	3.998	25.82	3.275
Buttocks	84.17	7.596	85.70 *†	7.318	82.05 *	7.315	81.29 †	7.907
Calf	33.41	2.910	33.74	2.838	32.85	2.967	33.08	3.003
Chest	81.85	7.465	83.34 †	7.215	80.04	7.076	78.20 †	7.896
Forearm	23.95	1.982	24.13 †	1.849	23.92 *	2.062	22.83 *†	2.198
Knee	34.47	2.531	34.71 †	2.472	34.37 *	2.544	33.25 *†	2.628
Shoulder	99.07	7.947	100.23	7.691	97.71	7.533	96.09	9.273
Thigh	49.99	5.867	50.52 †	5.738	49.49	5.882	47.95 †	6.146
Wrist	15.81	0.934	15.88 †	0.860	15.89 *	0.966	15.06 *†	0.981
Diameters (cm)								
Ankle	13.79	0.734	13.86 †	0.706	13.83 *	0.731	13.23 *†	0.681
Biacromial	36.53	2.577	36.78	2.418	36.25	2.763	35.94	2.682
Bi-iliac	25.59	2.018	26.25 *†	1.834	24.45 *	1.804	25.15 †	1.926
Bitrochanteric	29.63	2.317	30.25 *†	2.180	28.73 *	2.220	28.79 †	2.298
Chest	25.81	2.176	26.22 *†	2.081	25.21 *	2.139	25.14 †	2.336
Wrist	10.69	0.697	10.76 †	0.653	10.74 *	0.720	10.20 *†	0.714
Accessory Information								
Stature (dm)	16.61	0.868	16.84 †	0.837	16.41 *	0.807	15.96 *†	0.736
Lean body wt. (kg)	48.73	7.552	50.58 *†	7.305	46.41 *	6.971	45.07 †	7.668
Weight (kg)	55.79	12.212	57.96 †	12.487	53.31	10.779	50.42 †	12.338
% body fat	11.51	7.638	11.50	7.990	11.96	7.222	9.33	6.575
Age (years)	14.49	0.489	14.50	0.508	14.52	0.452	14.41	0.503

NOTE: Figures in parentheses represent number of subjects. Abdomen circumference represents the mean of upper and lower portions of the abdomen. Ankle, biceps, calf, forearm, knee, thigh and wrist circumferences represent the mean of the right and left sides. Ankle and wrist diameters represent the sum of the right and left sides.
* Significant differences (0.01 level), Caucasians vs. Negroes, Negroes vs. Orientals.
† Significant differences (0.01 level), Caucasians vs. Orientals.
** Age: 14.49.

TABLE VI

CIRCUMFERENCES, DIAMETERS AND ACCESSORY INFORMATION FOR ALL BOYS,
TENTH GRADE **

	All (454)		Caucasian (258)		Negro (152)		Oriental (36)	
	X̄	σ	X̄	σ	X̄	σ	X̄	σ
Circumferences (cm)								
Abdomen	71.07	7.164	72.20 *†	7.228	70.00 *	6.775	67.28 †	5.588
Ankle	22.00	1.520	22.34 *†	1.502	21.66 *	1.415	21.09 †	1.304
Biceps	28.60	2.943	28.50	2.847	29.19	2.953	26.99	2.731
Buttocks	87.14	6.843	88.25 *†	6.406	86.17 *	7.129	83.40 †	6.193
Calf	34.32	2.736	34.53	2.639	34.12	2.825	33.88	2.755
Chest	85.27	6.867	86.01 †	6.451	85.15	7.055	80.53 †	6.544
Forearm	25.02	1.841	25.07 †	1.692	25.32 *	1.949	23.61 *†	1.706
Knee	35.20	2.328	35.46 †	2.232	35.12 *	2.400	33.77 *†	2.112
Shoulder	103.99	7.293	104.41	7.041	104.23	7.275	100.42	7.751
Thigh	52.29	5.651	52.52 †	5.349	52.48	6.008	49.70 †	5.071
Wrist	16.17	0.808	16.23 †	0.749	16.29 *	0.793	15.34 *†	0.791
Diameters (cm)								
Ankle	14.18	0.693	14.24 †	0.646	14.24 *	0.681	13.57 *†	0.739
Biacromial	37.83	2.318	37.77	2.239	38.16	2.380	37.05	2.367
Bi-iliac	26.44	1.840	27.07 *†	1.687	25.57 *	1.705	25.88 †	1.694
Bitrochanteric	30.76	2.005	31.25 *†	1.865	30.19 *	1.973	29.81 †	2.078
Chest	26.74	1.908	27.06 *†	1.853	26.47 *	1.878	25.80 †	1.882
Wrist	11.04	0.616	11.05 †	0.577	11.16 *	0.601	10.50 *†	0.669
Accessory Information								
Stature (dm)	17.11	0.768	17.25 †	0.733	17.08 *	0.736	16.37 *†	0.656
Lean body wt. (kg)	53.15	6.808	54.48 *†	6.486	52.24 *	6.729	48.54 †	6.550
Weight (kg)	61.14	11.024	62.22 †	10.642	61.03	11.233	53.99 †	9.350
% body fat	12.12	7.548	11.58 *	7.374	13.37 *	7.662	9.38 *	6.017
Age (years)	15.32	0.489	15.27	0.487	15.42	0.482	15.19	0.464

NOTE: Figures in parentheses represent number of subjects. Abdomen circumference represents the
mean of upper and lower portions of the abdomen. Ankle, biceps, calf, forearm, knee, thigh and wrist
circumferences represent the mean of the right and left sides. Ankle and wrist diameters represent the
sum of the right and left sides.
* Significant differences (0.01 level), Caucasians vs. Negroes, Negroes vs. Orientals.
† Significant differences (0.01 level), Caucasians vs. Orientals.
** Age: 15.32.

Table VI (Cont'd.)

CIRCUMFERENCES, DIAMETERS AND ACCESSORY INFORMATION FOR ALL BOYS, ELEVENTH GRADE **

	All (466)		Caucasian (250)		Negro (168)		Oriental (37)	
	X̄	σ	X̄	σ	X̄	σ	X̄	σ
Circumferences (cm)								
Abdomen	72.50	7.161	73.89 *†	7.533	71.20 *	6.014	68.99 †	6.737
Ankle	22.18	1.508	22.54 *†	1.507	21.82 *	1.402	21.33 †	1.250
Biceps	29.75	2.746	29.59	2.792	30.31	2.545	28.24	2.680
Buttocks	88.66	6.390	90.13 *†	6.292	87.27 *	6.053	85.25 †	5.649
Calf	35.05	2.663	35.35	2.669	34.70	2.598	34.61	2.712
Chest	87.93	6.491	88.87 †	6.429	87.39	6.075	83.73 †	6.611
Forearm	25.76	1.726	25.85 †	1.667	25.95 *	1.714	24.32 *†	1.606
Knee	35.53	2.240	35.84 †	2.186	35.38 *	2.245	34.19 *†	2.050
Shoulder	107.11	6.625	107.38	6.668	107.40	6.257	103.66	7.177
Thigh	53.01	5.397	53.44 †	5.506	52.96	5.097	50.54 †	5.114
Wrist	16.38	0.789	16.48 †	0.748	16.44 *	0.764	15.51 *†	0.680
Diameters (cm)								
Ankle	14.17	0.721	14.25 †	0.697	14.20 *	0.705	13.58 *†	0.645
Biacromial	38.79	2.153	38.80	2.205	38.96	2.084	38.12	2.079
Bi-iliac	27.00	1.853	27.79 *†	1.720	25.97 *	1.523	26.42 †	1.645
Bitrochanteric	31.44	1.852	32.12 *†	1.751	30.71 *	1.643	30.44 †	1.488
Chest	27.33	1.908	27.76 *†	1.898	26.87 *	1.687	26.44 †	2.157
Wrist	11.25	0.614	11.29 †	0.599	11.33 *	0.590	10.66 *†	0.553
Accessory Information								
Stature (dm)	17.43	0.739	17.63 †	0.679	17.34 *	0.736	16.66 *†	0.501
Lean body wt. (kg)	56.05	6.592	58.01 *†	6.420	54.37 *	6.016	51.20 †	5.891
Weight (kg)	64.82	10.980	66.52 †	11.306	64.02	10.042	57.47 †	9.531
% body fat	12.66	7.363	11.87 *	7.451	14.31 *	6.970	10.05 *	7.033
Age (years)	16.36	0.508	16.30	0.468	16.46	0.546	16.25	0.507

NOTE: Figures in parentheses represent number of subjects. Abdomen circumference represents the mean of upper and lower portions of the abdomen. Ankle, biceps, calf, forearm, knee, thigh and wrist circumferences represent the mean of the right and left sides. Ankle and wrist diameters represent the sum of the right and left sides.
* Significant differences (0.01 level), Caucasians vs. Negroes, Negroes vs. Orientals.
† Significant differences (0.01 level), Caucasians vs. Orientals.
** Age: 16.36.

TABLE VII

CIRCUMFERENCES, DIAMETERS AND ACCESSORY INFORMATION FOR ALL BOYS, TWELFTH GRADE **

	All (403)		Caucasian (224)		Negro (140)		Oriental (35)	
	X̄	σ	X̄	σ	X̄	σ	X̄	σ
Circumferences (cm)								
Abdomen	74.18	7.480	75.50 *†	7.906	72.93 *	6.586	71.09 †	6.423
Ankle	22.08	1.417	22.37 *†	1.451	21.83 *	1.250	21.29 †	1.310
Biceps	30.72	2.848	30.46	2.774	31.58	2.788	29.20	2.614
Buttocks	90.26	6.578	91.56 *†	6.577	89.11 *	6.353	87.06 †	5.540
Calf	35.31	2.590	35.55	2.550	35.05	2.596	35.09	2.644
Chest	89.40	6.628	90.39 †	6.504	89.00	6.484	84.92 †	6.118
Forearm	26.37	1.733	26.36 †	1.588	26.77 *	1.790	24.94 *†	1.627
Knee	35.54	2.157	35.77 †	2.162	35.51	2.100	34.37 *†	1.954
Shoulder	109.35	6.429	109.34	6.384	110.26	6.210	106.26	6.737
Thigh	53.65	5.268	53.99 †	5.253	53.68	5.300	51.61 †	4.938
Wrist	16.56	0.807	16.61 †	0.758	16.71 *	0.758	15.67 *†	0.717
Diameters (cm)								
Ankle	14.31	0.747	14.36 †	0.727	14.38 *	0.695	13.77 *†	0.789
Biacromial	39.85	1.980	39.67	1.958	40.35	1.951	39.27	1.780
Bi-iliac	27.37	1.854	28.11 *†	1.754	26.36 *	1.473	26.91 †	1.715
Bitrochanteric	32.06	1.782	32.63 *†	1.693	31.43 *	1.638	31.06 †	1.604
Chest	27.94	1.804	28.30 *†	1.725	27.68 *	1.695	26.89 †	2.111
Wrist	11.36	0.617	11.37 †	0.583	11.49 *	0.573	10.77 *†	0.619
Accessory Information								
Stature (dm)	17.65	0.723	17.81 †	0.658	17.62 *	0.712	16.87 *†	0.587
Lean body wt. (kg)	58.71	6.474	60.25 *†	6.278	57.68 *	5.891	53.80 †	6.384
Weight (kg)	67.86	11.310	69.33 †	11.620	67.55	10.465	60.77 †	9.770
% body fat	12.60	7.338	12.16 *	7.463	13.75 *	7.317	10.76 *	6.137
Age (years)	17.29	0.450	17.23	0.418	17.41	0.474	17.19	0.455

NOTE: Figures in parentheses represent number of subjects. Abdomen circumference represents the mean of upper and lower portions of the abdomen. Ankle, biceps, calf, forearm, knee, thigh and wrist circumferences represent the mean of the right and left sides. Ankle and wrist diameters represent the sum of the right and left sides.
* Significant differences (0.01 level), Caucasians vs. Negroes, Negroes vs. Orientals.
† Significant differences (0.01 level), Caucasians vs. Orientals.
** Age: 17.29.

TABLE VIII

CIRCUMFERENCES, DIAMETERS AND ACCESSORY INFORMATION FOR ALL GIRLS,
NINTH GRADE **

	All (519)		Caucasian (316)		Negro (147)		Oriental (42)	
	$\bar{X}$	σ	$\bar{X}$	σ	$\bar{X}$	σ	$\bar{X}$	σ
Circumferences (cm)								
Abdomen	71.60	6.717	71.69 †	6.165	72.30 *	7.912	68.75 *†	5.588
Ankle	21.23	1.398	21.41 †	1.338	21.18	1.362	20.33 †	1.395
Biceps	26.15	2.593	26.18 †	2.428	26.59 *	2.770	24.64 *†	2.579
Buttocks	92.31	6.911	92.77 †	6.260	92.99 *	7.723	87.44 *†	6.675
Calf	34.22	2.689	34.43 †	2.583	34.25 *	2.724	33.01 *†	2.748
Chest	82.66	5.477	82.79 †	4.942	83.51 *	6.180	79.32 *†	5.549
Forearm	23.04	1.635	23.02 †	1.490	23.44 *	1.731	22.06 *†	1.694
Knee	35.01	2.460	34.87 †	2.322	35.71 *	2.563	33.74 *†	2.346
Shoulder	96.47	5.934	96.30	5.428	97.89 *	6.507	93.78 *†	6.165
Thigh	56.65	5.630	56.71 †	5.097	57.57 *	6.455	53.37 *†	5.033
Wrist	15.21	0.768	15.15 *†	0.700	15.56 *	0.760	14.59 *†	0.654
Diameters (cm)								
Ankle	12.25	0.625	12.27	0.579	12.33 *	0.665	11.88 *	0.663
Biacromial	35.23	1.792	35.17	1.695	35.70 *	1.864	34.47 *	1.780
Bi-iliac	26.24	1.798	26.57 *†	1.680	25.75 *	1.921	25.67 †	1.724
Bitrochanteric	30.79	1.894	31.02 †	1.772	30.63	2.107	29.75 †	1.662
Chest	25.22	1.587	25.35	1.509	25.17	1.703	24.62	1.604
Wrist	9.77	0.566	9.76	0.542	9.91	0.591	9.50	0.502
Accessory Information								
Stature (dm)	16.16	0.620	16.26 †	0.619	16.17 *	0.547	15.56 *†	0.448
Lean body wt. (kg)	45.30	5.351	45.98 †	5.085	45.33 *	5.552	41.37 *†	4.613
Weight (kg)	55.04	9.307	55.44 †	8.507	56.56 *	10.380	48.35 *†	7.871
% body fat	16.80	7.557	16.33 *	7.157	18.84 *	7.482	13.42 *	8.638
Age (years)	14.51	0.433	14.52	0.423	14.46	0.417	14.54	0.514

NOTE: Figures in parentheses represent number of subjects. Abdomen circumference represents the mean
of upper and lower portions of the abdomen. Ankle, biceps, calf, forearm, knee, thigh and wrist circumferences represent the mean of the right and left sides. Ankle and wrist diameters represent the sum of
the right and left sides.
* Significant differences (0.01 level), Caucasians vs. Negroes, Negroes vs. Orientals.
† Significant differences (0.01 level), Caucasians vs. Orientals.
** Age: 14.51.

TABLE IX

CIRCUMFERENCES, DIAMETERS AND ACCESSORY INFORMATION FOR ALL GIRLS,
TENTH GRADE **

	All (452)		Caucasian (268)		Negro (142)		Oriental (34)	
	X̄	σ	X̄	σ	X̄	σ	X̄	σ
Circumferences (cm)								
Abdomen	72.79	6.803	73.06 †	6.377	73.09 *	7.814	69.68 *†	5.074
Ankle	21.11	1.411	21.32 †	1.356	20.98	1.366	20.06 †	1.518
Biceps	26.15	2.605	26.16 †	2.514	26.52 *	2.640	24.65 *†	2.762
Buttocks	93.94	6.811	94.17 †	6.418	94.26 *	7.300	88.67 *†	6.062
Calf	34.31	2.678	34.56 †	2.623	34.21 *	2.648	32.93 *†	2.859
Chest	84.03	5.323	84.44 †	4.997	84.14 *	5.661	80.64 *†	5.339
Forearm	22.74	1.685	22.62 †	1.598	23.26 *	1.609	21.65 *†	1.998
Knee	36.13	2.584	36.19 †	2.485	36.42 *	2.728	34.47 *†	2.328
Shoulder	98.79	6.028	98.97	5.572	99.47 *	6.535	95.18 *	6.290
Thigh	57.00	5.238	57.15 †	4.885	57.62 *	5.696	53.80 *†	5.064
Wrist	15.06	0.822	14.97 *†	0.776	15.39 *	0.764	14.35 *†	0.826
Diameters (cm)								
Ankle	12.30	0.582	12.28	0.562	12.43*	0.571	11.90 *	0.606
Biacromial	35.81	1.815	35.74	1.757	36.24 *	1.811	34.83 *	1.692
Bi-iliac	26.84	1.859	27.29 *†	1.761	26.14 *	1.932	26.14 †	1.187
Bitrochanteric	30.97	1.811	31.27 †	1.802	30.68	1.804	29.81 †	1.301
Chest	25.43	1.585	25.49	1.522	25.54	1.686	24.62 †	1.523
Wrist	9.98	0.573	9.91	0.538	10.22	0.544	9.51	0.533
Accessory Information								
Stature (dm)	16.29	0.622	16.37 †	0.611	16.31 *	0.550	15.56 *†	0.505
Lean body wt. (kg)	46.83	5.386	47.51 †	5.052	46.86 *	5.343	41.84 *†	4.170
Weight (kg)	56.57	9.474	56.83 †	8.724	58.03 *	10.459	49.23 *†	7.938
% body fat	16.33	7.664	15.66 *	7.397	18.26 *	7.317	13.85	9.648
Age (years)	15.24	0.432	15.20	0.346	15.31	0.518	15.12	0.503

NOTE: Figures in parentheses represent number of subjects. Abdomen circumference represents the mean
of upper and lower portions of the abdomen. Ankle, biceps, calf, forearm, knee, thigh and wrist circumferences represent the mean of the right and left sides. Ankle and wrist diameters represent the sum of
the right and left sides.
* Significant differences (0.01 level), Caucasians vs. Negroes, Negroes vs. Orientals.
† Significant differences (0.01 level), Caucasians vs. Orientals.
** Age: 15.24.

TABLE X

CIRCUMFERENCES, DIAMETERS AND ACCESSORY INFORMATION FOR ALL GIRLS, ELEVENTH GRADE **

	All (424)		Caucasian (246)		Negro (139)		Oriental (36)	
	X̄	σ	X̄	σ	X̄	σ	X̄	σ
Circumferences (cm)								
Abdomen	69.80	6.510	69.91 †	6.042	70.35 *	7.388	66.81 *†	5.223
Ankle	21.27	1.373	21.50 †	1.317	21.08	1.358	20.42 †	1.361
Biceps	26.84	2.591	26.92 †	2.452	27.01 *	2.753	25.56 *†	2.617
Buttocks	93.56	6.535	94.34 †	5.907	93.51 *	7.236	88.65 *†	5.773
Calf	34.73	2.560	35.05 †	2.420	34.49	2.627	33.51 †	2.785
Chest	83.53	5.216	83.94 †	4.776	83.55 *	5.686	80.59 *†	5.457
Forearm	23.05	1.586	22.95 †	1.484	23.46 *	1.625	22.16 *†	1.689
Knee	36.08	2.470	36.17 †	2.367	36.31 *	2.544	34.54 *†	2.396
Shoulder	98.16	6.211	97.98	5.763	99.12 *	5.820	95.76 *	6.105
Thigh	57.39	4.948	57.76 †	4.420	57.53 *	6.631	54.34 *†	4.668
Wrist	15.27	0.750	15.22 *†	0.716	15.51 *	0.727	14.63 *†	0.637
Diameters (cm)								
Ankle	12.19	0.604	12.14	0.562	12.35 *	0.633	11.91 *	0.584
Biacromial	35.80	1.713	35.70	1.626	36.25 *	1.756	34.74 *	1.598
Bi-iliac	26.85	1.735	27.43 *†	1.540	25.90 *	1.713	26.67 †	1.415
Bitrochanteric	30.98	1.715	31.30 †	1.623	30.68	1.838	30.14 †	1.285
Chest	24.47	1.420	24.63	1.381	24.30	1.455	24.10	1.441
Wrist	9.65	0.525	9.58	0.510	9.83	0.509	9.39	0.469
Accessory Information								
Stature (dm)	16.35	0.620	16.45 †	0.617	16.34 *	0.538	15.71 *†	0.509
Lean body wt. (kg)	46.07	5.083	46.92 †	4.998	45.64 *	4.996	42.34 *†	3.931
Weight (kg)	57.09	9.243	57.65 †	8.552	57.98 *	10.108	50.07 *†	7.496
% body fat	18.45	7.554	17.93 *	7.032	20.33 *	7.303	14.34 *	9.707
Age (years)	16.23	0.378	16.21	0.346	16.27	0.395	16.16	0.441

NOTE: Figures in parentheses represent number of subjects. Abdomen circumference represents the mean of upper and lower portions of the abdomen. Ankle, biceps, calf, forearm, knee, thigh and wrist circumferences represent the mean of the right and left sides. Ankle and wrist diameters represent the sum of the right and left sides.
* Significant differences (0.01 level), Caucasians vs. Negroes, Negroes vs. Orientals.
† Significant differences (0.01 level), Caucasians vs. Orientals.
** Age: 16.23.

TABLE XI

CIRCUMFERENCES, DIAMETERS AND ACCESSORY INFORMATION FOR ALL GIRLS, TWELFTH GRADE **

	All (404)		Caucasian (245)		Negro (117)		Oriental (37)	
	X̄	σ	X̄	σ	X̄	σ	X̄	σ
Circumferences (cm)								
Abdomen	72.77	7.184	72.92	6.686	73.25	8.133	70.22	6.723
Ankle	21.35	1.433	21.57 †	1.379	21.20	1.384	20.57 †	1.565
Biceps	26.84	2.785	26.88	2.733	27.11	2.788	25.78	2.883
Buttocks	94.49	7.202	94.95 †	6.701	95.09 *	7.994	89.99 *†	6.274
Calf	34.95	2.762	35.19 †	2.677	34.85	2.792	33.81 †	2.894
Chest	84.68	5.530	84.91 †	5.264	84.98 *	5.847	81.99 *†	5.637
Forearm	23.59	1.661	23.53 †	1.592	24.03 *	1.615	22.72 *†	1.797
Knee	36.36	2.800	36.34 †	2.703	36.86 *	2.920	34.94 *†	2.586
Shoulder	99.00	6.024	98.98	5.863	99.83 *	6.142	96.52 *	6.132
Thigh	56.25	5.554	56.39 †	5.121	57.13 *	6.067	52.77 *†	5.422
Wrist	15.22	0.811	15.19 *†	0.774	15.51 *	0.814	14.57 *†	0.610
Diameters (cm)								
Ankle	12.55	0.615	12.54	0.587	12.72 *	0.628	12.16 *	0.518
Biacromial	35.80	1.826	35.78	1.751	36.15 *	1.952	35.07 *	1.630
Bi-iliac	27.66	1.889	28.15 *†	1.718	26.82 *	1.937	27.26 †	1.790
Bitrochanteric	31.42	1.899	31.67 †	1.827	31.24	2.025	30.54 †	1.622
Chest	24.57	1.532	24.71	1.529	24.45	1.513	24.06	1.539
Wrist	10.04	0.546	10.02	0.528	10.22	0.545	9.62	0.359
Accessory Information								
Stature (dm)	16.38	0.641	16.50 †	0.623	16.39 *	0.561	15.70 *†	0.499
Lean body wt. (kg)	47.62	5.742	48.51 †	5.632	47.32 *	5.675	43.44 *†	4.441
Weight (kg)	57.91	10.139	58.21 †	9.542	59.60 *	11.020	51.20 *†	8.489
% body fat	16.84	7.944	15.86 *	7.626	19.63 *	7.378	14.02 *	9.258
Age (years)	17.23	0.390	17.23	0.351	17.23	0.411	17.19	0.462

NOTE: Figures in parentheses represent number of subjects. Abdomen circumference represents the mean of upper and lower portions of the abdomen. Ankle, biceps, calf, forearm, knee, thigh and wrist circumferences represent the mean of the right and left sides. Ankle and wrist diameters represent the sum of the right and left sides.
* Significant differences (0.01 level), Caucasians vs. Negroes, Negroes vs. Orientals.
† Significant differences (0.01 level), Caucasians vs. Orientals.
** Age: 17.23.

DEVELOPMENT OF SIMPLIFIED
METHOD BY USE OF REGRESSION
EQUATIONS

IN AN EFFORT TO DEVELOP an even more simplified method for determining body composition, we subjected our body measurement data to regression analyses. This simpler method should be one that could be easily used in the public schools.

In order to identify the adolescent who may be becoming obese it is necessary to measure changes in body composition in addition to changes in body height and weight during growth. Changes in total weight could then be separated into two components: changes in amount of body fat and changes in lean body weight.

Ninety-one boys and 97 girls in our subsample were measured anthropometrically and densiometrically. These adolescents were approximately sixteen years old.

The parameters used in the development of the regression equations for estimating lean body weight were the six extremity circumferences (biceps, forearm, wrist, knee, calf, and ankle), height and weight.

Anthropometric and density measurements were done using the method already described.

We limited our regression parameters to those measurements that would require neither the use of special equipment (other than a centimeter tape measure) nor the removal of clothing. (Facilities for measuring height and weight are available in most public schools.) We excluded the diameter measurements because they require the use of an anthropometer. We also excluded trunk circumferences as these measurements necessitate clothing removal on the part of the subject.

Linear regressions of measured lean body weight on the six extremity circumferences, height, and weight were determined for four groups: Caucasian and Oriental boys, Negro boys, Caucasian and Oriental girls, Negro girls. Various transformations (linear, logarithm, square, cube, square root) of the six circumferences, height, and weight were investigated for each sex, and each race within each sex. Those combinations of transformations resulting in the highest correlation coefficients were used in the regression equations.

All data analyses were done by computer.

Means, standard deviations, and ranges for all anthropometric measurements and other parameters for all subjects by sex and race within sex are given in Tables XII, XIII, XIV, and XV.

Table XVI shows the means, standard deviations and ranges for all subjects, for measured lean body weight (underwater weighing) by sex and race.

Two- and three-variable regression equations are presented in Table XVII, as are the multiple correlation coefficients between measured lean body weight and estimated lean body weight. In these equations weight is measured and estimated in kilograms, height is measured in decimeters, and circumferences are measured in tenths of centimeters. The circumference value used is the mean of right and left extremities. A single regression equation is given for Caucasians and Orientals because our anthropometric analyses indicate that skeletal frames for the Negroes differ from those of the other two races. Statistical tests were made to determine if two, or possibly all three races, could be combined in one regression equation for the estimation of lean body weight. Each pair of races was examined and the calculated F statistic compared with the tabulated F statistic. The generated F statistic for the boys indicated (5 percent level) that Caucasian and Oriental boys could be combined in a single regression equation, and that a separate equation was needed for the Negro boys. This confirmed the results of earlier analyses of anthropometric measurements. Generated F statistic of pairwise racial comparisons for the girls did not indicate statistically significant differences among the races at the 5 percent level.

The regression equations were developed specifically for the estimation of lean body weight. A lower correlation coefficient ($r = 0.5$–0.6) was found between measured percent of fat (underwater weighing) and percent of fat as derived from estimated lean body weights, than was found for measured versus estimated lean body weight. There is no fixed total body weight associated with a specific measured lean body weight (underwater weighing), and a small change in lean body weight causes a proportionately larger change in percent of body fat.

Two- and three-way lean body weight estimation tables have been developed from each of the regression equations.

Since these tables have not been tested by use on a different group of teenagers, we do not suggest that they be employed at this time to estimate lean body weight. Also they are based on relatively small numbers of individuals, particularly those for the Negro boys and girls. For these reasons, we are including in the appendix only the samples of the two- and three-way tables that apply to the Caucasian and Oriental boys. These are intended, not for use, but to illustrate the way regression equations could be developed so that they would have practical applications for assessing changes in lean body weight and body composition during growth.

TABLE XII

MEANS, STANDARD DEVIATIONS AND RANGES OF CIRCUMFERENCES, DIAMETERS AND ACCESSORY INFORMATION FOR 91 ADOLESCENT BOYS CLASSIFIED BY RACE

	All Boys (N = 91)			Caucasian Boys (N = 55)			Negro Boys (N = 25)			Oriental Boys (N = 11)		
	X̄	σ	100% Range	X̄	σ	100% Range	X̄	σ	100% Range	X̄	σ	100% Range
Circumferences (cm)												
Upper abdomen	72.93	7.966	59.20– 99.80	72.85	7.900	59.20– 98.20	75.18	8.455	62.50– 99.80	68.24	4.107	63.50– 76.90
Lower abdomen	74.76	9.150	60.70–105.20	75.05	9.316	60.70–105.00	76.61	9.361	62.90–105.20	69.12	4.427	64.50– 78.50
Abdomen*	73.85	8.526	59.95–102.50	73.95	8.570	59.95–101.60	75.89	8.893	62.70–102.50	68.68	4.257	64.00– 77.70
Ankle **	22.30	1.662	18.65– 26.75	22.30	1.602	18.65– 26.75	22.73	1.748	19.15– 25.50	21.31	1.291	19.00– 23.65
Biceps **	29.68	3.555	21.90– 39.20	29.24	3.427	21.90– 38.95	31.37	3.571	24.75– 39.20	28.01	2.572	24.65– 32.55
Buttocks **	90.27	7.913	75.30–113.00	90.29	7.348	77.90–111.00	92.18	9.146	75.30–113.00	85.82	5.456	77.00– 93.60
Calf **	35.27	3.239	27.85– 43.10	34.85	3.090	29.75– 43.00	36.26	3.733	27.85– 43.10	35.08	2.049	31.30– 37.30
Chest	88.56	7.313	73.10–109.10	88.08	7.120	73.10–108.60	91.51	7.437	79.20–109.10	84.30	4.908	77.30– 93.00
Forearm **	25.80	2.143	20.50– 30.55	25.60	1.933	20.50– 30.30	26.90	2.291	22.45– 30.55	24.32	1.497	22.15– 26.95
Knee **	36.25	2.631	31.30– 44.45	35.99	2.277	32.05– 42.65	37.47	3.037	32.50– 44.45	34.79	2.124	31.30– 37.50
Shoulder	106.75	7.633	87.50–129.20	106.05	7.375	87.50–126.00	110.10	7.441	96.90–129.20	102.65	6.282	93.40–113.40
Thigh **	53.77	6.902	41.75– 76.65	53.08	6.505	41.75– 70.30	56.71	7.602	44.25– 76.65	50.50	4.288	43.15– 58.00
Wrist **	16.39	0.835	14.35– 18.50	16.41	0.689	14.60– 18.50	16.73	0.860	15.15– 18.20	15.49	0.801	14.35– 17.10

* Mean of upper and lower abdomen. (It is necessary to measure the abdomen at two levels in order to describe adequately size and change in shape as fatness develops. The average is taken because in both male and female it is the same fractional part of the total of the eleven circumferences.)
** Mean of right and left sides.

TABLE XIII

BOYS

	All Boys (N = 91)			Caucasian Boys (N = 55)			Negro Boys (N = 25)			Oriental Boys (N = 11)		
	X̄	σ	100% Range	X̄	σ	100% Range	X̄	σ	100% Range	X̄	σ	100% Range
Diameters (cm)												
Ankle ***	13.91	0.761	12.20– 16.00	13.86	0.645	12.20– 15.60	14.28	0.697	13.00– 16.00	13.31	0.966	12.20–15.50
Biacromial	38.08	2.177	31.80– 43.00	37.86	2.248	31.80– 42.60	38.86	1.750	35.40– 43.00	37.39	2.207	34.20–41.00
Bi-iliac	27.10	1.882	22.70– 31.30	27.49	1.775	24.20– 31.30	26.46	1.918	22.70– 30.20	26.60	1.807	24.50–30.20
Bitrochanteric	31.59	1.966	27.00– 36.10	31.85	1.929	27.80– 36.10	31.41	1.966	27.00– 34.00	30.68	1.828	28.50–34.10
Chest	27.32	1.617	23.20– 30.90	27.41	1.541	23.80– 30.30	27.50	1.760	23.20– 30.90	26.51	1.398	24.10–29.40
Wrist ***	11.14	0.634	9.20– 12.50	11.15	0.539	9.20– 12.10	11.39	0.629	10.00– 12.50	10.55	0.699	9.60–12.10
Accessory Information												
Stature (dm)	17.35	0.754	15.12– 19.15	17.40	0.635	16.04– 19.15	17.54	0.818	15.12– 19.00	16.62	0.728	15.85–18.33
Lean body wt. calculated (kg)	55.19	6.485	39.24– 68.69	55.65	6.269	41.55– 68.69	56.14	5.955	39.24– 67.33	50.69	6.891	41.40–65.78
Weight (kg)	65.55	13.120	42.10–105.10	64.70	12.453	42.10–105.10	71.20	13.635	42.20–102.70	56.95	8.721	44.10–72.10
% Body fat	14.16	10.030	−8.03– 43.20	12.52	9.525	−8.03– 35.16	19.39	10.364	1.25– 43.20	10.47	6.718	0.63–25.80
Age (years)	15.99	0.430	15.01– 17.54	15.97	0.467	15.01– 17.54	16.05	0.375	15.39– 17.19	15.92	0.322	15.49–16.41

*** Sum of right and left sides.

TABLE XIV

MEANS, STANDARD DEVIATIONS AND RANGES OF CIRCUMFERENCES, DIAMETERS AND ACCESSORY INFORMATION FOR 97 ADOLESCENT GIRLS CLASSIFIED BY RACE

	All Girls (N = 97)			Caucasian Girls (N = 62)			Negro Girls (N = 26)			Oriental Girls (N = 9)		
	X̄	σ	100% Range	X̄	σ	100% Range	X̄	σ	100% Range	X̄	σ	100% Range
Circumferences (cm)												
Upper abdomen	66.76	6.705	56.90–101.50	66.36	5.931	56.90–101.50	68.62	8.534	59.70– 94.20	64.12	3.711	58.60– 71.80
Lower abdomen	79.74	8.623	63.60–121.10	80.52	7.477	68.80–121.10	79.37	11.347	63.60–112.00	75.39	4.568	70.30– 85.10
Abdomen*	73.25	7.487	61.65–111.30	73.44	6.553	62.85–111.30	74.00	9.835	61.65–103.10	69.75	3.836	64.45– 78.45
Ankle**	21.22	1.488	17.70– 25.20	21.44	1.435	18.70– 25.20	21.04	1.582	18.45– 25.00	20.21	1.007	17.70– 21.65
Biceps**	26.83	2.962	20.30– 39.30	26.79	2.639	22.25– 39.30	27.63	3.445	22.25– 37.75	24.85	2.558	20.30– 29.10
Buttocks**	94.56	6.648	80.60–119.50	94.88	5.334	84.00–117.20	95.79	8.604	82.20–119.50	88.82	5.327	80.60– 98.90
Calf**	34.74	3.008	28.30– 44.60	35.07	2.721	28.90– 42.95	34.62	3.640	28.30– 44.60	32.85	1.973	28.35– 34.95
Chest	84.50	5.395	71.10–109.30	84.72	4.742	74.50–109.30	85.68	6.131	74.20–103.80	79.55	4.622	71.10– 87.50
Forearm**	23.31	1.871	18.80– 30.35	23.12	1.651	19.60– 30.35	24.21	2.011	20.55– 29.70	22.02	1.729	18.80– 24.80
Knee**	35.91	2.698	30.15– 46.90	35.90	2.390	30.15– 43.95	36.49	3.377	31.00– 46.90	34.30	1.617	31.50– 37.05
Shoulder	98.72	5.553	85.60–123.60	98.52	4.951	88.40–123.60	100.61	6.459	85.60–118.90	94.57	3.879	86.50–100.70
Thigh**	57.62	5.363	45.90– 76.65	57.67	4.494	46.90– 71.30	58.84	6.803	45.90– 76.65	53.69	4.174	46.45– 60.00
Wrist**	15.30	0.769	13.60– 18.00	15.24	0.715	13.60– 17.95	15.66	0.789	14.45– 18.00	14.62	0.438	13.85– 15.15

* Mean of upper and lower abdomen. (It is necessary to measure the abdomen at two levels in order to describe adequately size and change in shape as fatness develops. The average is taken because in both male and female it is the same fractional part of the total of the eleven circumferences.)
** Mean of right and left sides.

TABLE XV

GIRLS

	All Girls (N = 97)			Caucasian Girls (N = 62)			Negro Girls (N = 26)			Oriental Girls (N = 9)		
	X̄	σ	100% Range	X̄	σ	100% Range	X̄	σ	100% Range	X̄	σ	100% Range
Diameters (cm)												
Ankle ***	12.22	0.559	10.70– 14.10	12.20	0.546	10.70– 14.10	12.34	0.559	11.50– 13.70	11.97	0.548	11.30–12.80
Biacromial	36.04	1.772	32.20– 41.80	36.02	1.832	32.20– 41.80	36.30	1.652	32.50– 39.90	35.42	1.499	32.90–37.60
Bi-iliac	27.07	1.684	23.30– 32.60	27.38	1.561	23.30– 32.50	26.59	1.915	23.30– 32.60	26.38	1.187	24.80–28.30
Bitrochanteric	31.32	1.726	27.90– 36.80	31.57	1.612	27.90– 35.70	31.01	2.014	27.90– 36.80	30.44	0.998	28.80–31.70
Chest	25.75	1.665	21.50– 32.80	25.74	1.500	22.80– 31.90	26.13	2.051	21.50– 32.80	24.78	0.937	23.10–26.40
Wrist ***	9.68	0.518	8.70– 11.70	9.60	0.494	8.70– 10.80	9.99	0.489	9.00– 11.70	9.37	0.310	8.80– 9.80
Accessory Information												
Stature (dm)	16.37	0.623	14.90– 17.85	16.47	0.642	15.15– 17.85	16.31	0.449	15.63– 17.23	15.81	0.604	14.90–16.83
Lean body wt. calculated (kg)	47.56	5.442	36.45– 66.27	48.15	5.349	36.45– 64.74	47.59	5.723	37.45– 66.27	43.43	2.819	39.76–47.92
Weight (kg)	56.86	10.127	39.10– 102.50	56.96	8.619	40.50–102.50	59.52	12.884	41.80–100.90	48.48	4.821	39.10–57.00
% body fat	15.40	8.902	-1.96– 40.39	14.75	8.013	-1.00– 36.84	18.92	9.489	0.84– 40.39	9.70	8.969	-1.96–25.67
Age (years)	15.95	0.373	15.08– 17.65	16.00	0.393	15.08– 17.65	15.92	0.321	15.38– 16.77	15.69	0.231	15.27–15.93

*** Sum of right and left sides.

TABLE XVI

MEANS, STANDARD DEVIATIONS AND RANGES OF MEASURED LEAN
BODY WEIGHT—UNDERWATER WEIGHING—(KG) FOR 188
ADOLESCENTS CLASSIFIED BY SEX AND RACE

		Boys				Girls		
	N	X̄	σ	100% Range	N	X̄	σ	100% Range
All	91	56.07	8.703	36.00–75.73	97	41.40	6.212	28.55–65.18
Caucasian	55	55.46	8.220	36.00–74.29	62	41.49	6.001	28.55–65.18
Negro	25	59.69	9.159	40.16–75.73	26	42.73	6.750	33.93–61.81
Oriental	11	50.89	6.291	41.47–61.68	9	36.98	3.397	30.83–42.34

TABLE XVII

TWO- AND THREE-VARIABLE REGRESSION EQUATIONS AND MULTIPLE CORRELATIONS BY SEX/RACIAL GROUPS

	Number of Variables	Estimated Lean Body Weight (kg)	Multiple Correlation with Measured Lean Body Weight (kg)
Boys			
Caucasian and Oriental	2	$\log_e$ Lean Body Weight = 1.109 $\log_e$ Weight* − 0.000008 Knee³ −0.234	0.926
	3	$\log_e$ Lean Body Weight = 1.099 $\log_e$ Weight − 0.000008 Knee³ +0.000005 Wrist³ −0.214	0.942
Negro	2	$\log_e$ Lean Body Weight = 1.311 $\log_e$ Weight − 0.00001 Knee³ −0.879	0.893
	3	$\log_e$ Lean Body Weight = 1.020 $\log_e$ Weight − 0.00001 Knee³ +0.00009 Wrist³ −0.107	0.929
Girls			
Caucasian and Oriental	2	Lean Body Weight³ = 16.415 Height³ +0.229 Weight³ −42786.6	0.858
	3	Lean Body Weight³ = 16.894 Height³ +0.197 Weight³ +0.494 Calf² −60116.2	0.868
Negro	2	Lean Body Weight³ = 17.858 Height³ +0.200 Weight³ −43212.1	0.918
	3	Lean Body Weight³ = 19.748 Height³ +0.092 Weight³ +1.571 Calf² −92173.9	0.939

* Weight in kilograms; height in decimeters; circumferences in centimeters.

TABLE XVIII

CAUCASIAN AND ORIENTAL BOYS, LEAN BODY WEIGHT

Weight (kg)	30	31	32	33	34	35	36	37	38	39	40	41	42	43
						Knee (cm)								
40	37.8	37.0	36.1	35.3	34.3	33.4	32.4	31.4	30.4	29.4	28.3	27.3	26.2	25.1
41	38.8	38.0	37.1	36.2	35.3	34.3	33.3	32.3	31.3	30.2	29.1	28.0	26.9	25.8
42	39.9	39.0	38.1	37.2	36.2	35.2	34.2	33.2	32.1	31.0	29.9	28.8	27.6	26.5
43	40.9	40.0	39.1	38.2	37.2	36.2	35.1	34.0	32.9	31.8	30.7	29.5	28.4	27.2
44	42.0	41.1	40.1	39.1	38.1	37.1	36.0	34.9	33.8	32.6	31.5	30.3	29.1	27.9
45	43.0	42.1	41.1	40.1	39.1	38.0	36.9	35.8	34.6	33.5	32.3	31.0	29.8	28.6
46	44.1	43.1	42.1	41.1	40.0	38.9	37.8	36.7	35.5	34.3	33.0	31.8	30.5	29.3
47	45.1	44.2	43.1	42.1	41.0	39.9	38.7	37.5	36.3	35.1	33.8	32.6	31.3	30.0
48	46.2	45.2	44.2	43.1	42.0	40.8	39.6	38.4	37.2	35.9	34.6	33.3	32.0	30.7
49	47.2	46.2	45.2	44.1	42.9	41.7	40.5	39.3	38.0	36.7	35.4	34.1	32.7	31.4
50	48.3	47.3	46.2	45.1	43.9	42.7	41.4	40.2	38.9	37.6	36.2	34.9	33.5	32.1
51	49.4	48.3	47.2	46.0	44.9	43.6	42.4	41.1	39.7	38.4	37.0	35.6	34.2	32.8
52	50.4	49.3	48.2	47.0	45.8	44.6	43.3	42.0	40.6	39.2	37.8	36.4	35.0	33.5
53	51.5	50.4	49.2	48.0	46.8	45.5	44.2	42.8	41.5	40.0	38.6	37.2	35.7	34.2
54	52.6	51.4	50.3	49.0	47.8	46.5	45.1	43.7	42.3	40.9	39.4	37.9	36.4	34.9
55	53.6	52.5	51.3	50.0	48.7	47.4	46.0	44.6	43.2	41.7	40.2	38.7	37.2	35.6
56	54.7	53.5	52.3	51.0	49.7	48.4	46.9	45.5	44.0	42.5	41.0	39.5	37.9	36.4
57	55.8	54.6	53.3	52.0	50.7	49.3	47.9	46.4	44.9	43.4	41.8	40.3	38.7	37.1
58	56.9	55.6	54.4	53.0	51.7	50.3	48.8	47.3	45.8	44.2	42.6	41.0	39.4	37.8
59	57.9	56.7	55.4	54.0	52.7	51.2	49.7	48.2	46.6	45.1	43.4	41.8	40.2	38.5
60	59.0	57.8	56.4	55.1	53.6	52.2	50.6	49.1	47.5	45.9	44.3	42.6	40.9	39.2
61	60.1	58.8	57.5	56.1	54.6	53.1	51.6	50.0	48.4	46.7	45.1	43.4	41.7	39.9
62	61.2	59.9	58.5	57.1	55.6	54.1	52.5	50.9	49.3	47.6	45.9	44.2	42.4	40.7
63	62.3	60.9	59.5	58.1	56.6	55.0	53.4	51.8	50.1	48.4	46.7	44.9	43.2	41.4
64	63.4	62.0	60.6	59.1	57.6	56.0	54.4	52.7	51.0	49.3	47.5	45.7	43.9	42.1
65	64.5	63.1	61.6	60.1	58.6	57.0	55.3	53.6	51.9	50.1	48.3	46.5	44.7	42.8
66	65.5	64.1	62.7	61.1	59.6	57.9	56.2	54.5	52.8	51.0	49.1	47.3	45.4	43.6
67	66.6	65.2	63.7	62.2	60.5	58.9	57.2	55.4	53.6	51.8	50.0	48.1	46.2	44.3
68	67.7	66.3	64.8	63.2	61.5	59.9	58.1	56.3	54.5	52.7	50.8	48.9	46.9	45.0
69	68.8	67.3	65.8	64.2	62.5	60.8	59.1	57.3	55.4	53.5	51.6	49.7	47.7	45.7
70	69.9	68.4	66.9	65.2	63.5	61.8	60.0	58.2	56.3	54.4	52.4	50.5	48.5	46.5
71	71.0	69.5	67.9	66.2	64.5	62.8	60.9	59.1	57.2	55.2	53.3	51.3	49.2	47.2
72	72.1	70.6	69.0	67.3	65.5	63.7	61.9	60.0	58.1	56.1	54.1	52.0	50.0	47.9
73	73.2	71.6	70.0	68.3	66.5	64.7	62.8	60.9	58.9	56.9	54.9	52.8	50.8	48.7
74	74.3	72.7	71.1	69.3	67.5	65.7	63.8	61.8	59.8	57.8	55.7	53.6	51.5	49.4
75	75.4	73.8	72.1	70.4	68.5	66.7	64.7	62.8	60.7	58.7	56.6	54.4	52.3	50.1
76	76.5	74.9	73.2	71.4	69.5	67.6	65.7	63.7	61.6	59.5	57.4	55.2	53.1	50.9
77	77.6	76.0	74.2	72.4	70.6	68.6	66.6	64.6	62.5	60.4	58.2	56.0	53.8	51.6
78	78.8	77.1	75.3	73.5	71.6	69.6	67.6	65.5	63.4	61.2	59.1	56.8	54.6	52.3
79	79.9	78.2	76.4	74.5	72.6	70.6	68.5	66.4	64.3	62.1	59.9	57.6	55.4	53.1
80	81.0	79.2	77.4	75.5	73.6	71.6	69.5	67.4	65.2	63.0	60.7	58.4	56.1	53.8
81	82.1	80.3	78.5	76.6	74.6	72.6	70.4	68.3	66.1	63.8	61.6	59.2	56.9	54.6
82	83.2	81.4	79.6	77.6	75.6	73.5	71.4	69.2	67.0	64.7	62.4	60.0	57.7	55.3
83	84.3	82.5	80.6	78.7	76.6	74.5	72.4	70.1	67.9	65.6	63.2	60.9	58.5	56.0
84	85.4	83.6	81.7	79.7	77.6	75.5	73.3	71.1	68.8	66.4	64.1	61.7	59.2	56.8
85	86.6	84.7	82.8	80.7	78.7	76.5	74.3	72.0	69.7	67.3	64.9	62.5	60.0	57.5
86	87.7	85.8	83.8	81.8	79.7	77.5	75.2	72.9	70.6	68.2	65.7	63.3	60.8	58.3
87	88.8	86.9	84.9	82.8	80.7	78.5	76.2	73.9	71.5	69.1	66.6	64.1	61.6	59.0
88	89.9	88.0	86.0	83.9	81.7	79.5	77.2	74.8	72.4	69.9	67.4	64.9	62.3	59.8
89	91.0	89.1	87.1	84.9	82.7	80.5	78.1	75.7	73.3	70.8	68.3	65.7	63.1	60.5
90	92.2	90.2	88.1	86.0	83.8	81.5	79.1	76.7	74.2	71.7	69.1	66.5	63.9	61.3
91	93.3	91.3	89.2	87.0	84.8	82.5	80.1	77.6	75.1	72.6	70.0	67.3	64.7	62.0
92	94.4	92.4	90.3	88.1	85.8	83.5	81.0	78.6	76.0	73.4	70.8	68.1	65.5	62.8
93	95.6	93.5	91.4	89.1	86.8	84.5	82.0	79.5	76.9	74.3	71.7	69.0	66.2	63.5
94	96.7	94.6	92.4	90.2	87.9	85.5	83.0	80.4	77.8	75.2	72.5	69.8	67.0	64.3
95	97.8	95.7	93.5	91.2	88.9	86.5	83.9	81.4	78.7	76.1	73.3	70.6	67.8	65.0
96	99.0	96.8	94.6	92.3	89.9	87.5	84.9	82.3	79.7	76.9	74.2	71.4	68.6	65.8
97	100.1	97.9	95.7	93.4	90.9	88.5	85.9	83.3	80.6	77.8	75.0	72.2	69.4	66.5
98	101.2	99.0	96.8	94.4	92.0	89.5	86.9	84.2	81.5	78.7	75.9	73.0	70.2	67.3
99	102.4	100.2	97.9	95.5	93.0	90.5	87.8	85.1	82.4	79.6	76.7	73.9	71.0	68.0
100	103.5	101.3	99.0	96.5	94.0	91.5	88.8	86.1	83.3	80.5	77.6	74.7	71.7	68.8
101	104.6	102.4	100.0	97.6	95.1	92.5	89.8	87.0	84.2	81.4	78.5	75.5	72.5	69.5
102	105.8	103.5	101.1	98.7	96.1	93.5	90.8	88.0	85.1	82.3	79.3	76.3	73.3	70.3
103	106.9	104.6	102.2	99.7	97.2	94.5	91.7	88.9	86.1	83.1	80.2	77.2	74.1	71.1
104	108.1	105.7	103.3	100.8	98.2	95.5	92.7	89.9	87.0	84.0	81.0	78.0	74.9	71.8
105	109.2	106.9	104.4	101.9	99.2	96.5	93.7	90.8	87.9	84.9	81.9	78.8	75.7	72.6
106	110.3	108.0	105.5	102.9	100.3	97.5	94.7	91.8	88.8	85.8	82.7	79.6	76.5	73.3
107	111.5	109.1	106.6	104.0	101.3	98.5	95.7	92.7	89.7	86.7	83.6	80.5	77.3	74.1
108	112.6	110.2	107.7	105.1	102.3	99.5	96.7	93.7	90.7	87.6	84.5	81.3	78.1	74.9
109	113.8	111.3	108.8	106.1	103.4	100.6	97.6	94.7	91.6	88.5	85.3	82.1	78.9	75.6
110	114.9	112.5	109.9	107.2	104.4	101.6	98.6	95.6	92.5	89.4	86.2	82.9	79.7	76.4

TABLE XIX

CAUCASIAN AND ORIENTAL BOYS, LEAN BODY WEIGHT

Wrist: 14.0 cm

Weight (kg)	30	31	32	33	34	35	Knee (cm) 36	37	38	39	40	41	42	43
40	38.3	37.5	36.6	35.8	34.8	33.9	32.9	31.9	30.9	29.8	28.7	27.7	26.6	25.5
41	39.4	38.5	37.7	36.7	35.8	34.8	33.8	32.8	31.7	30.6	29.5	28.4	27.3	26.2
42	40.4	39.6	38.7	37.7	36.7	35.7	34.7	33.6	32.6	31.4	30.3	29.2	28.0	26.9
43	41.5	40.6	39.7	38.7	37.7	36.7	35.6	34.5	33.4	32.3	31.1	29.9	28.8	27.6
44	42.6	41.6	40.7	39.7	38.7	37.6	36.5	35.4	34.3	33.1	31.9	30.7	29.5	28.3
45	43.6	42.7	41.7	40.7	39.6	38.6	37.4	36.3	35.1	33.9	32.7	31.5	30.2	29.0
46	44.7	43.7	42.7	41.7	40.6	39.5	38.4	37.2	36.0	34.8	33.5	32.3	31.0	29.7
47	45.8	44.8	43.8	42.7	41.6	40.4	39.3	38.1	36.8	35.6	34.3	33.0	31.7	30.4
48	46.8	45.8	44.8	43.7	42.6	41.4	40.2	39.0	37.7	36.4	35.1	33.8	32.5	31.1
49	47.9	46.9	45.8	44.7	43.5	42.3	41.1	39.9	38.6	37.3	35.9	34.6	33.2	31.8
50	49.0	47.9	46.8	45.7	44.5	43.3	42.0	40.7	39.4	38.1	36.7	35.3	34.0	32.6
51	50.1	49.0	47.9	46.7	45.5	44.2	43.0	41.6	40.3	38.9	37.5	36.1	34.7	33.3
52	51.1	50.0	48.9	47.7	46.5	45.2	43.9	42.5	41.2	39.8	38.3	36.9	35.5	34.0
53	52.2	51.1	49.9	48.7	47.5	46.2	44.8	43.4	42.0	40.6	39.2	37.7	36.2	34.7
54	53.3	52.2	51.0	49.7	48.4	47.1	45.7	44.3	42.9	41.5	40.0	38.5	37.0	35.4
55	54.4	53.2	52.0	50.7	49.4	48.1	46.7	45.3	43.8	42.3	40.8	39.3	37.7	36.2
56	55.5	54.3	53.0	51.8	50.4	49.0	47.6	46.2	44.7	43.1	41.6	40.0	38.5	36.9
57	56.6	55.4	54.1	52.8	51.4	50.0	48.6	47.1	45.5	44.0	42.4	40.8	39.2	37.6
58	57.7	56.4	55.1	53.8	52.4	51.0	49.5	48.0	46.4	44.8	43.2	41.6	40.0	38.3
59	58.8	57.5	56.2	54.8	53.4	51.9	50.4	48.9	47.3	45.7	44.1	42.4	40.7	39.1
60	59.9	58.6	57.2	55.8	54.4	52.9	51.4	49.8	48.2	46.5	44.9	43.2	41.5	39.8
61	61.0	59.6	58.3	56.9	55.4	53.9	52.3	50.7	49.1	47.4	45.7	44.0	42.3	40.5
62	62.1	60.7	59.3	57.9	56.4	54.8	53.3	51.6	50.0	48.3	46.5	44.8	43.0	41.2
63	63.2	61.8	60.4	58.9	57.4	55.8	54.2	52.5	50.8	49.1	47.4	45.6	43.8	42.0
64	64.3	62.9	61.4	59.9	58.4	56.8	55.1	53.5	51.7	50.0	48.2	46.4	44.5	42.7
65	65.4	64.0	62.5	61.0	59.4	57.8	56.1	54.4	52.6	50.8	49.0	47.2	45.3	43.4
66	66.5	65.0	63.6	62.0	60.4	58.7	57.0	55.3	53.5	51.7	49.8	48.0	46.1	44.2
67	67.6	66.1	64.6	63.0	61.4	59.7	58.0	56.2	54.4	52.6	50.7	48.8	46.8	44.9
68	68.7	67.2	65.7	64.1	62.4	60.7	58.9	57.1	55.3	53.4	51.5	49.6	47.6	45.6
69	69.8	68.3	66.7	65.1	63.4	61.7	59.9	58.1	56.2	54.3	52.3	50.4	48.4	46.4
70	70.9	69.4	67.8	66.1	64.4	62.7	60.9	59.0	57.1	55.1	53.2	51.2	49.2	47.1

TABLE XX

CAUCASIAN AND ORIENTAL BOYS, LEAN BODY WEIGHT

Wrist: 14.5 cm

Weight (kg)	30	31	32	33	34	35	Knee (cm) 36	37	38	39	40	41	42	43
40	38.4	37.6	36.7	35.8	34.9	33.9	32.9	31.9	30.9	29.9	28.8	27.7	26.6	25.5
41	39.4	38.6	37.7	36.8	35.8	34.9	33.8	32.8	31.8	30.7	29.6	28.5	27.3	26.2
42	40.5	39.6	38.7	37.8	36.8	35.8	34.8	33.7	32.6	31.5	30.4	29.2	28.1	26.9
43	41.6	40.7	39.7	38.8	37.8	36.7	35.7	34.5	33.4	32.3	31.2	30.0	28.8	27.6
44	42.6	41.7	40.8	39.8	38.7	37.7	36.6	35.5	34.3	33.1	32.0	30.8	29.6	28.3
45	43.7	42.8	41.8	40.8	39.7	38.6	37.5	36.3	35.2	34.0	32.8	31.5	30.3	29.0
46	44.8	43.8	42.8	41.8	40.7	39.6	38.4	37.2	36.0	34.8	33.6	32.3	31.0	29.7
47	45.8	44.8	43.8	42.8	41.6	40.5	39.3	38.1	36.9	35.6	34.4	33.1	31.8	30.5
48	46.9	45.9	44.8	43.8	42.6	41.5	40.3	39.0	37.8	36.5	35.2	33.9	32.5	31.2
49	48.0	47.0	45.9	44.8	43.6	42.4	41.2	39.9	38.6	37.3	36.0	34.6	33.3	31.9
50	49.1	48.0	46.9	45.8	44.6	43.4	42.1	40.8	39.5	38.2	36.8	35.4	34.0	32.6
51	50.1	49.1	47.9	46.8	45.6	44.3	43.0	41.7	40.4	39.0	37.6	36.2	34.8	33.3
52	51.2	50.1	49.0	47.8	46.5	45.3	44.0	42.6	41.2	39.8	38.4	37.0	35.5	34.0
53	52.3	51.2	50.0	48.8	47.5	46.2	44.9	43.5	42.1	40.7	39.2	37.7	36.3	34.8
54	53.4	52.2	51.0	49.8	48.5	47.2	45.8	44.4	43.0	41.5	40.0	38.5	37.0	35.5
55	54.5	53.3	52.1	50.8	49.5	48.2	46.8	45.3	43.9	42.4	40.9	39.3	37.8	36.2
56	55.6	54.4	53.1	51.8	50.5	49.1	47.7	46.2	44.7	43.2	41.7	40.1	38.5	36.9
57	56.7	55.4	54.2	52.9	51.5	50.1	48.6	47.1	45.6	44.1	42.5	40.9	39.3	37.7
58	57.8	56.5	55.2	53.9	52.5	51.0	49.6	48.0	46.5	44.9	43.3	41.7	40.0	38.4
59	58.9	57.6	56.3	54.9	53.5	52.0	50.5	49.0	47.4	45.8	44.1	42.5	40.8	39.1
60	60.0	58.7	57.3	55.9	54.5	53.0	51.4	49.9	48.3	46.6	45.0	43.3	41.6	39.8
61	61.0	59.7	58.4	56.9	55.5	54.0	52.4	50.8	49.1	47.5	45.8	44.1	42.3	40.6
62	62.2	60.8	59.4	58.0	56.5	54.9	53.3	51.7	50.0	48.3	46.6	44.9	43.1	41.3
63	63.3	61.9	60.5	59.0	57.5	55.9	54.3	52.6	50.9	49.2	47.4	45.6	43.8	42.0
64	64.4	63.0	61.5	60.0	58.5	56.9	55.2	53.5	51.8	50.0	48.3	46.4	44.6	42.8
65	65.5	64.1	62.6	61.1	59.5	57.9	56.2	54.5	52.7	50.9	49.1	47.2	45.4	43.5
66	66.6	65.1	63.7	62.1	60.5	58.8	57.1	55.4	53.6	51.8	49.9	48.0	46.1	44.2
67	67.7	66.2	64.7	63.1	61.5	59.8	58.1	56.3	54.5	52.6	50.8	48.8	46.9	45.0
68	68.8	67.3	65.8	64.2	62.5	60.8	59.0	57.2	55.4	53.5	51.6	49.6	47.7	45.7
69	69.9	68.4	66.8	65.2	63.5	61.8	60.0	58.2	56.3	54.4	52.4	50.4	48.5	46.5
70	71.0	69.5	67.9	66.3	64.5	62.8	60.9	59.1	57.2	55.2	53.3	51.3	49.2	47.2

TABLE XXI

CAUCASIAN AND ORIENTAL BOYS, LEAN BODY WEIGHT

Wrist: 15.0 cm

Weight (kg)	30	31	32	33	34	35	Knee (cm) 36	37	38	39	40	41	42	43
40	38.5	37.6	36.8	35.9	34.9	34.0	33.0	32.0	31.0	29.9	28.8	27.7	26.7	25.6
41	39.5	38.7	37.8	36.9	35.9	34.9	33.9	32.9	31.8	30.7	29.6	28.5	27.4	26.3
42	40.6	39.7	38.8	37.8	36.9	35.9	34.8	33.8	32.7	31.5	30.4	29.3	28.1	27.0
43	41.6	40.7	39.8	38.8	37.8	36.8	35.7	34.6	33.5	32.4	31.2	30.0	28.9	27.7
44	42.7	41.8	40.8	39.8	38.8	37.7	36.6	35.5	34.4	33.2	32.0	30.8	29.6	28.4
45	43.8	42.8	41.8	40.8	39.8	38.7	37.6	36.4	35.2	34.0	32.8	31.6	30.3	29.1
46	44.8	43.9	42.9	41.8	40.7	39.6	38.5	37.3	36.1	34.9	33.6	32.4	31.1	29.8
47	45.9	44.9	43.9	42.8	41.7	40.6	39.4	38.2	37.0	35.7	34.4	33.1	31.8	30.5
48	47.0	46.0	44.9	43.8	42.7	41.5	40.3	39.1	37.8	36.5	35.2	33.9	32.6	31.2
49	48.1	47.0	46.0	44.8	43.7	42.5	41.2	40.0	38.7	37.4	36.0	34.7	33.3	31.9
50	49.1	48.1	47.0	45.8	44.7	43.4	42.2	40.9	39.6	38.2	36.8	35.5	34.1	32.7
51	50.2	49.1	48.0	46.9	45.6	44.4	43.1	41.8	40.4	39.1	37.7	36.2	34.8	33.4
52	51.3	50.2	49.1	47.9	46.6	45.3	44.0	42.7	41.3	39.9	38.5	37.0	35.6	34.1
53	52.4	51.3	50.1	48.9	47.6	46.3	45.0	43.6	42.2	40.7	39.3	37.8	36.3	34.8
54	53.5	52.3	51.1	49.9	48.6	47.3	45.9	44.5	43.1	41.6	40.1	38.6	37.1	35.5
55	54.6	53.4	52.2	50.9	49.6	48.2	46.8	45.4	43.9	42.4	40.9	39.4	37.8	36.3
56	55.7	54.5	53.2	51.9	50.6	49.2	47.8	46.3	44.8	43.3	41.7	40.2	38.6	37.0
57	56.8	55.5	54.3	52.9	51.6	50.2	48.7	47.2	45.7	44.1	42.6	41.0	39.3	37.7
58	57.9	56.6	55.3	54.0	52.6	51.1	49.6	48.1	46.6	45.0	43.4	41.8	40.1	38.4
59	59.0	57.7	56.4	55.0	53.6	52.1	50.6	49.0	47.5	45.8	44.2	42.5	40.9	39.2
60	60.1	58.8	57.4	56.0	54.6	53.1	51.5	50.0	48.3	46.7	45.0	43.3	41.6	39.9
61	61.2	59.8	58.5	57.0	55.6	54.0	52.5	50.9	49.2	47.6	45.9	44.1	42.4	40.6
62	62.3	60.9	59.5	58.1	56.6	55.0	53.4	51.8	50.1	48.4	46.7	44.9	43.2	41.4
63	63.4	62.0	60.6	59.1	57.6	56.0	54.4	52.7	51.0	49.3	47.5	45.7	43.9	42.1
64	64.5	63.1	61.6	60.1	58.6	57.0	55.3	53.6	51.9	50.1	48.3	46.5	44.7	42.8
65	65.6	64.2	62.7	61.2	59.6	58.0	56.3	54.6	52.8	51.0	49.2	47.3	45.5	43.6
66	66.7	65.3	63.8	62.2	60.6	58.9	57.2	55.5	53.7	51.9	50.0	48.1	46.2	44.3
67	67.8	66.3	64.8	63.2	61.6	59.9	58.2	56.4	54.6	52.7	50.8	48.9	47.0	45.1
68	68.9	67.4	65.9	64.3	62.6	60.9	59.1	57.3	55.5	53.6	51.7	49.7	47.8	45.8
69	70.0	68.5	67.0	65.3	63.6	61.9	60.1	58.3	56.4	54.5	52.5	50.5	48.5	46.5
70	71.1	69.6	68.0	66.4	64.6	62.9	61.1	59.2	57.3	55.3	53.3	51.3	49.3	47.3

TABLE XXII

CAUCASIAN AND ORIENTAL BOYS, LEAN BODY WEIGHT

Wrist: 15.5 cm

Weight (kg)	30	31	32	33	34	35	Knee (cm) 36	37	38	39	40	41	42	43
40	38.5	37.7	36.8	35.9	35.0	34.0	33.1	32.0	31.0	30.0	28.9	27.8	26.7	25.6
41	39.6	38.7	37.8	36.9	36.0	35.0	34.0	32.9	31.9	30.8	29.7	28.6	27.4	26.3
42	40.6	39.8	38.9	37.9	36.9	35.9	34.9	33.8	32.7	31.6	30.5	29.3	28.2	27.0
43	41.7	40.8	39.9	38.9	37.9	36.9	35.8	34.7	33.6	32.4	31.3	30.1	28.9	27.7
44	42.8	41.9	40.9	39.9	38.9	37.8	36.7	35.6	34.4	33.3	32.1	30.9	29.7	28.4
45	43.8	42.9	41.9	40.9	39.8	38.8	37.6	36.5	35.3	34.1	32.9	31.6	30.4	29.1
46	44.9	44.0	42.9	41.9	40.8	39.7	38.5	37.4	36.2	34.9	33.7	32.4	31.1	29.9
47	46.0	45.0	44.0	42.9	41.8	40.6	39.5	38.3	37.0	35.8	34.5	33.2	31.9	30.6
48	47.1	46.1	45.0	43.9	42.8	41.6	40.4	39.2	37.9	36.6	35.3	34.0	32.6	31.3
49	48.1	47.1	46.0	44.9	43.8	42.6	41.3	40.1	38.8	37.4	36.1	34.7	33.4	32.0
50	49.2	48.2	47.1	45.9	44.7	43.5	42.2	41.0	39.6	38.3	36.9	35.5	34.1	32.7
51	50.3	49.2	48.1	46.9	45.7	44.5	43.2	41.9	40.5	39.1	37.7	36.3	34.9	33.4
52	51.4	50.3	49.1	47.9	46.7	45.4	44.1	42.8	41.4	40.0	38.5	37.1	35.6	34.2
53	52.5	51.4	50.2	49.0	47.7	46.4	45.0	43.7	42.3	40.8	39.4	37.9	36.4	34.9
54	53.6	52.4	51.2	50.0	48.7	47.4	46.0	44.6	43.1	41.7	40.2	38.7	37.1	35.6
55	54.7	53.5	52.3	51.0	49.7	48.3	46.9	45.5	44.0	42.5	41.0	39.5	37.9	36.3
56	55.8	54.6	53.3	52.0	50.7	49.3	47.9	46.4	44.9	43.4	41.8	40.2	38.7	37.1
57	56.9	55.6	54.4	53.0	51.7	50.3	48.8	47.3	45.8	44.2	42.6	41.0	39.4	37.8
58	58.0	56.7	55.4	54.1	52.7	51.2	49.7	48.2	46.7	45.1	43.5	41.8	40.2	38.5
59	59.1	57.8	56.5	55.1	53.7	52.2	50.7	49.1	47.5	45.9	44.3	42.6	40.9	39.2
60	60.2	58.9	57.5	56.1	54.7	53.2	51.6	50.0	48.4	46.8	45.1	43.4	41.7	40.0
61	61.3	59.9	58.6	57.1	55.7	54.1	52.6	51.0	49.3	47.6	45.9	44.2	42.5	40.7
62	62.4	61.0	59.6	58.2	56.7	55.1	53.5	51.9	50.2	48.5	46.8	45.0	43.2	41.4
63	63.5	62.1	60.7	59.2	57.7	56.1	54.5	52.8	51.1	49.4	47.6	45.8	44.0	42.2
64	64.6	63.2	61.7	60.2	58.7	57.1	55.4	53.7	52.0	50.2	48.4	46.6	44.8	42.9
65	65.7	64.3	62.8	61.3	59.7	58.1	56.4	54.6	52.9	51.1	49.3	47.4	45.5	43.7
66	66.8	65.4	63.9	62.3	60.7	59.0	57.3	55.6	53.8	51.9	50.1	48.2	46.3	44.4
67	67.9	66.5	64.9	63.4	61.7	60.0	58.3	56.5	54.7	52.8	50.9	49.0	47.1	45.1
68	69.0	67.6	66.0	64.4	62.7	61.0	59.2	57.4	55.6	53.7	51.8	49.8	47.9	45.9
69	70.2	68.6	67.1	65.4	63.7	62.0	60.2	58.4	56.5	54.6	52.6	50.6	48.6	46.6
70	71.3	69.7	68.1	66.5	64.8	63.0	61.2	59.3	57.4	55.4	53.4	51.4	49.4	47.4
71	72.4	70.8	69.2	67.5	65.8	64.0	62.1	60.2	58.3	56.3	54.3	52.2	50.2	48.1
72	73.5	71.9	70.3	68.6	66.8	65.0	63.1	61.2	59.2	57.2	55.1	53.0	51.0	48.9
73	74.6	73.0	71.4	69.6	67.8	66.0	64.0	62.1	60.1	58.0	56.0	53.9	51.7	49.6
74	75.8	74.1	72.4	70.7	68.8	67.0	65.0	63.0	61.0	58.9	56.8	54.7	52.5	50.3
75	76.9	75.2	73.5	71.7	69.9	68.0	66.0	64.0	61.9	59.8	57.7	55.5	53.3	51.1
76	78.0	76.3	74.6	72.8	70.9	68.9	66.9	64.9	62.8	60.7	58.5	56.3	54.1	51.8
77	79.1	77.4	75.7	73.8	71.9	69.9	67.9	65.8	63.7	61.5	59.3	57.1	54.9	52.6
78	80.3	78.5	76.7	74.9	72.9	70.9	68.9	66.8	64.6	62.4	60.2	57.9	55.6	53.3
79	81.4	79.7	77.8	75.9	74.0	71.9	69.9	67.7	65.5	63.3	61.0	58.7	56.4	54.1
80	82.5	80.8	78.9	77.0	75.0	72.9	70.8	68.7	66.4	64.2	61.9	59.6	57.2	54.9
81	83.7	81.9	80.0	78.1	76.0	74.0	71.8	69.6	67.4	65.1	62.7	60.4	58.0	55.6
82	84.8	83.0	81.1	79.1	77.1	75.0	72.8	70.6	68.3	66.0	63.6	61.2	58.8	56.4
83	85.9	84.1	82.2	80.2	78.1	76.0	73.8	71.5	69.2	66.8	64.4	62.0	59.6	57.1
84	87.1	85.2	83.3	81.2	79.1	77.0	74.7	72.4	70.1	67.7	65.3	62.8	60.4	57.9
85	88.2	86.3	84.4	82.3	80.2	78.0	75.7	73.4	71.0	68.6	66.2	63.7	61.2	58.6
86	89.4	87.4	85.4	83.4	81.2	79.0	76.7	74.3	71.9	69.5	67.0	64.5	62.0	59.4
87	90.5	88.6	86.5	84.4	82.2	80.0	77.7	75.3	72.9	70.4	67.9	65.3	62.7	60.2
88	91.7	89.7	87.6	85.5	83.3	81.0	78.7	76.2	73.8	71.3	68.7	66.1	63.5	60.9
89	92.8	90.8	88.7	86.6	84.3	82.0	79.6	77.2	74.7	72.2	69.6	67.0	64.3	61.7
90	94.0	91.9	89.8	87.6	85.4	83.0	80.6	78.2	75.6	73.1	70.4	67.8	65.1	62.4
91	95.1	93.1	90.9	88.7	86.4	84.0	81.6	79.1	76.6	74.0	71.3	68.6	65.9	63.2
92	96.2	94.2	92.0	89.8	87.5	85.1	82.6	80.1	77.5	74.8	72.2	69.5	66.7	64.0

TABLE XXIII

CAUCASIAN AND ORIENTAL BOYS, LEAN BODY WEIGHT

Wrist: 16.0 cm

Weight (kg)	30	31	32	33	34	35	Knee (cm) 36	37	38	39	40	41	42	43
40	38.6	37.8	36.9	36.0	35.1	34.1	33.1	32.1	31.1	30.0	28.9	27.9	26.8	25.6
41	39.7	38.8	37.9	37.0	36.0	35.0	34.0	33.0	31.9	30.8	29.7	28.6	27.5	26.4
42	40.7	39.8	38.9	38.0	37.0	36.0	34.9	33.9	32.8	31.7	30.5	29.4	28.2	27.1
43	41.8	40.9	40.0	39.0	38.0	36.9	35.9	34.8	33.6	32.5	31.3	30.2	29.0	27.8
44	42.9	41.9	41.0	40.0	38.9	37.9	36.8	35.7	34.5	33.3	32.1	30.9	29.7	28.5
45	43.9	43.0	42.0	41.0	39.9	38.8	37.7	36.5	35.4	34.2	32.9	31.7	30.5	29.2
46	45.0	44.0	43.0	42.0	40.9	39.8	38.6	37.4	36.2	35.0	33.7	32.5	31.2	29.9
47	46.1	45.1	44.1	43.0	41.9	40.7	39.5	38.3	37.1	35.8	34.6	33.3	31.9	30.6
48	47.2	46.1	45.1	44.0	42.9	41.7	40.5	39.2	38.0	36.7	35.4	34.0	32.7	31.3
49	48.2	47.2	46.1	45.0	43.8	42.6	41.4	40.1	38.8	37.5	36.2	34.8	33.4	32.1
50	49.3	48.3	47.2	46.0	44.8	43.6	42.3	41.0	39.7	38.4	37.0	35.6	34.2	32.8
51	50.4	49.3	48.2	47.0	45.8	44.6	43.3	41.9	40.6	39.2	37.8	36.4	34.9	33.5
52	51.5	50.4	49.2	48.0	46.8	45.5	44.2	42.8	41.5	40.0	38.6	37.2	35.7	34.2
53	52.6	51.5	50.3	49.1	47.8	46.5	45.1	43.7	42.3	40.9	39.4	38.0	36.5	34.9
54	53.7	52.5	51.3	50.1	48.8	47.4	46.1	44.7	43.2	41.7	40.3	38.7	37.2	35.7
55	54.8	53.6	52.4	51.1	49.8	48.4	47.0	45.6	44.1	42.6	41.1	39.5	38.0	36.4
56	55.9	54.7	53.4	52.1	50.8	49.4	47.9	46.5	45.0	43.4	41.9	40.3	38.7	37.1
57	57.0	55.7	54.5	53.1	51.8	50.3	48.9	47.4	45.9	44.3	42.7	41.1	39.5	37.9
58	58.1	56.8	55.5	54.2	52.8	51.3	49.8	48.3	46.7	45.2	43.5	41.9	40.3	38.6
59	59.2	57.9	56.6	55.2	53.8	52.3	50.8	49.2	47.6	46.0	44.4	42.7	41.0	39.3
60	60.3	59.0	57.6	56.2	54.8	53.3	51.7	50.1	48.5	46.9	45.2	43.5	41.8	40.1
61	61.4	60.1	58.7	57.3	55.8	54.2	52.7	51.1	49.4	47.7	46.0	44.3	42.5	40.8
62	62.5	61.1	59.7	58.3	56.8	55.2	53.6	52.0	50.3	48.6	46.9	45.1	43.3	41.5
63	63.6	62.2	60.8	59.3	57.8	56.2	54.6	52.9	51.2	49.5	47.7	45.9	44.1	42.3
64	64.7	63.3	61.9	60.4	58.8	57.2	55.5	53.8	52.1	50.3	48.5	46.7	44.9	43.0
65	65.8	64.4	62.9	61.4	59.8	58.2	56.5	54.8	53.0	51.2	49.4	47.5	45.6	43.7
66	66.9	65.5	64.0	62.4	60.8	59.2	57.4	55.7	53.9	52.0	50.2	48.3	46.4	44.5
67	68.0	66.6	65.1	63.5	61.8	60.1	58.4	56.6	54.8	52.9	51.0	49.1	47.2	45.2
68	69.2	67.7	66.1	64.5	62.9	61.1	59.4	57.5	55.7	53.8	51.9	49.9	47.9	46.0
69	70.3	68.8	67.2	65.6	63.9	62.1	60.3	58.5	56.6	54.7	52.7	50.7	48.7	46.7
70	71.4	69.9	68.3	66.6	64.9	63.1	61.3	59.4	57.5	55.5	53.5	51.5	49.5	47.5
71	72.5	71.0	69.3	67.7	65.9	64.1	62.2	60.3	58.4	56.4	54.4	52.3	50.3	48.2
72	73.7	72.1	70.4	68.7	66.9	65.1	63.2	61.3	59.3	57.3	55.2	53.2	51.1	48.9
73	74.8	73.2	71.5	69.8	67.9	66.1	64.2	62.2	60.2	58.1	56.1	54.0	51.8	49.7
74	75.9	74.3	72.6	70.8	69.0	67.1	65.1	63.1	61.1	59.0	56.9	54.8	52.6	50.4
75	77.0	75.4	73.7	71.9	70.0	68.1	66.1	64.1	62.0	59.9	57.8	55.6	53.4	51.2
76	78.2	76.5	74.7	72.9	71.0	69.1	67.1	65.0	62.9	60.8	58.6	56.4	54.2	51.9
77	79.3	77.6	75.8	74.0	72.1	70.1	68.0	66.0	63.8	61.7	59.5	57.2	55.0	52.7
78	80.4	78.7	76.9	75.0	73.1	71.1	69.0	66.9	64.7	62.5	60.3	58.0	55.8	53.5
79	81.6	79.8	78.0	76.1	74.1	72.1	70.0	67.8	65.7	63.4	61.2	58.9	56.5	54.2
80	82.7	80.9	79.1	77.1	75.1	73.1	71.0	68.8	66.6	64.3	62.0	59.7	57.3	55.0
81	83.8	82.0	80.2	78.2	76.2	74.1	71.9	69.7	67.5	65.2	62.9	60.5	58.1	55.7
82	85.0	83.1	81.2	79.3	77.2	75.1	72.9	70.7	68.4	66.1	63.7	61.3	58.9	56.5
83	86.1	84.3	82.3	80.3	78.3	76.1	73.9	71.6	69.3	67.0	64.6	62.1	59.7	57.2
84	87.3	85.4	83.4	81.4	79.3	77.1	74.9	72.6	70.2	67.9	65.4	63.0	60.5	58.0
85	88.4	86.5	84.5	82.5	80.3	78.1	75.9	73.5	71.2	68.7	66.3	63.8	61.3	58.7
86	89.5	87.6	85.6	83.5	81.4	79.1	76.8	74.5	72.1	69.6	67.1	64.6	62.1	59.5
87	90.7	88.7	86.7	84.6	82.4	80.1	77.8	75.4	73.0	70.5	68.0	65.4	62.9	60.3
88	91.8	89.9	87.8	85.7	83.4	81.2	78.8	76.4	73.9	71.4	68.9	66.3	63.7	61.0
89	93.0	91.0	88.9	86.7	84.5	82.2	79.8	77.3	74.9	72.3	69.7	67.1	64.5	61.8
90	94.1	92.1	90.0	87.8	85.5	83.2	80.8	78.3	75.8	73.2	70.6	67.9	65.3	62.6
91	95.3	93.2	91.1	88.9	86.6	84.2	81.8	79.3	76.7	74.1	71.4	68.8	66.0	63.3
92	96.4	94.4	92.2	90.0	87.6	85.2	82.8	80.2	77.6	75.0	72.3	69.6	66.8	64.1

TABLE XXIV

CAUCASIAN AND ORIENTAL BOYS, LEAN BODY WEIGHT

Wrist: 16.5 cm

Weight (kg)	30	31	32	33	34	35	*Knee* (cm) 36	37	38	39	40	41	42	43
40	38.7	37.8	37.0	36.1	35.1	34.2	33.2	32.2	31.1	30.1	29.0	27.9	26.8	25.7
41	39.7	38.9	38.0	37.1	36.1	35.1	34.1	33.1	32.0	30.9	29.8	28.7	27.5	26.4
42	40.8	39.9	39.0	38.1	37.1	36.1	35.0	33.9	32.8	31.7	30.6	29.4	28.3	27.1
43	41.9	41.0	40.0	39.1	38.1	37.0	35.9	34.8	33.7	32.6	31.4	30.2	29.0	27.8
44	42.9	42.0	41.1	40.1	39.0	38.0	36.9	35.7	34.6	33.4	32.2	31.0	29.8	28.5
45	44.0	43.1	42.1	41.1	40.0	38.9	37.8	36.6	35.4	34.2	33.0	31.8	30.5	29.3
46	45.1	44.1	43.1	42.1	41.0	39.9	38.7	37.5	36.3	35.1	33.8	32.5	31.3	30.0
47	46.2	45.2	44.1	43.1	42.0	40.8	39.6	38.4	37.2	35.9	34.6	33.3	32.0	30.7
48	47.3	46.2	45.2	44.1	42.9	41.8	40.6	39.3	38.0	36.7	35.4	34.1	32.8	31.4
49	48.3	47.3	46.2	45.1	43.9	42.7	41.5	40.2	38.9	37.6	36.2	34.9	33.5	32.1
50	49.4	48.4	47.3	46.1	44.9	43.7	42.4	41.1	39.8	38.4	37.1	35.7	34.3	32.8
51	50.5	49.4	48.3	47.1	45.9	44.6	43.3	42.0	40.7	39.3	37.9	36.5	35.0	33.6
52	51.6	50.5	49.3	48.1	46.9	45.6	44.3	42.9	41.5	40.1	38.7	37.2	35.8	34.3
53	52.7	51.6	50.4	49.2	47.9	46.6	45.2	43.8	42.4	41.0	39.5	38.0	36.5	35.0
54	53.8	52.6	51.4	50.2	48.9	47.5	46.2	44.7	43.3	41.8	40.3	38.8	37.3	35.7
55	54.9	53.7	52.5	51.2	49.9	48.5	47.1	45.7	44.2	42.7	41.2	39.6	38.0	36.5
56	56.0	54.8	53.5	52.2	50.9	49.5	48.0	46.6	45.1	43.5	42.0	40.4	38.8	37.2
57	57.1	55.9	54.6	53.2	51.9	50.5	49.0	47.5	46.0	44.4	42.8	41.2	39.6	37.9
58	58.2	56.9	55.6	54.3	52.9	51.4	49.9	48.4	46.8	45.2	43.6	42.0	40.3	38.7
59	59.3	58.0	56.7	55.3	53.9	52.4	50.9	49.3	47.7	46.1	44.5	42.8	41.1	39.4
60	60.4	59.1	57.7	56.3	54.9	53.4	51.8	50.2	48.6	47.0	45.3	43.6	41.9	40.1
61	61.5	60.2	58.8	57.4	55.9	54.4	52.8	51.2	49.5	47.8	46.1	44.4	42.6	40.9
62	62.6	61.3	59.9	58.4	56.9	55.3	53.7	52.1	50.4	48.7	46.9	45.2	43.4	41.6
63	63.7	62.4	60.9	59.4	57.9	56.3	54.7	53.0	51.3	49.6	47.8	46.0	44.2	42.4
64	64.8	63.4	62.0	60.5	58.9	57.3	55.6	53.9	52.2	50.4	48.6	46.8	44.9	43.1
65	66.0	64.5	63.1	61.5	59.9	58.3	56.6	54.9	53.1	51.3	49.5	47.6	45.7	43.8
66	67.1	65.6	64.1	62.6	60.9	59.3	57.6	55.8	54.0	52.2	50.3	48.4	46.5	44.6
67	68.2	66.7	65.2	63.6	62.0	60.3	58.5	56.7	54.9	53.0	51.1	49.2	47.3	45.3
68	69.3	67.8	66.3	64.6	63.0	61.3	59.5	57.7	55.8	53.9	52.0	50.0	48.0	46.1
69	70.4	68.9	67.3	65.7	64.0	62.2	60.4	58.6	56.7	54.8	52.8	50.8	48.8	46.8
70	71.6	70.0	68.4	66.7	65.0	63.2	61.4	59.5	57.6	55.6	53.7	51.6	49.6	47.6
71	72.7	71.1	69.5	67.8	66.0	64.2	62.4	60.5	58.5	56.5	54.5	52.4	50.4	48.3
72	73.8	72.2	70.6	68.8	67.1	65.2	63.3	61.4	59.4	57.4	55.3	53.3	51.2	49.0
73	74.9	73.3	71.6	69.9	68.1	66.2	64.3	62.3	60.3	58.3	56.2	54.1	51.9	49.8
74	76.1	74.4	72.7	70.9	69.1	67.2	65.3	63.3	61.2	59.1	57.0	54.9	52.7	50.5
75	77.2	75.5	73.8	72.0	70.1	68.2	66.2	64.2	62.1	60.0	57.9	55.7	53.5	51.3
76	78.3	76.6	74.9	73.1	71.2	69.2	67.2	65.2	63.0	60.9	58.7	56.5	54.3	52.1
77	79.5	77.7	76.0	74.1	72.2	70.2	68.2	66.1	64.0	61.8	59.6	57.3	55.1	52.8
78	80.6	78.9	77.1	75.2	73.2	71.2	69.2	67.0	64.9	62.7	60.4	58.2	55.9	53.6
79	81.7	80.0	78.1	76.2	74.3	72.2	70.1	68.0	65.8	63.6	61.3	59.0	56.7	54.3
80	82.9	81.1	79.2	77.3	75.3	73.2	71.1	69.0	66.7	64.4	62.1	59.8	57.4	55.1
81	84.0	82.2	80.3	78.4	76.3	74.2	72.1	69.9	67.6	65.3	63.0	60.6	58.2	55.8
82	85.1	83.3	81.4	79.4	77.4	75.3	73.1	70.8	68.5	66.2	63.8	61.4	59.0	56.6
83	86.3	84.4	82.5	80.5	78.4	76.3	74.0	71.8	69.5	67.1	64.7	62.3	59.8	57.3
84	87.4	85.6	83.6	81.6	79.4	77.3	75.0	72.7	70.4	68.0	65.6	63.1	60.6	58.1
85	88.6	86.7	84.7	82.6	80.5	78.3	76.0	73.7	71.3	68.9	66.4	63.9	61.4	58.9
86	89.7	87.8	85.8	83.7	81.5	79.3	77.0	74.6	72.2	69.8	67.3	64.7	62.2	59.6
87	90.9	88.9	86.9	84.8	82.6	80.3	78.0	75.6	73.2	70.7	68.1	65.6	63.0	60.4
88	92.0	90.0	88.0	85.8	83.6	81.3	79.0	76.5	74.1	71.6	69.0	66.4	63.8	61.2
89	93.2	91.2	89.1	86.9	84.7	82.3	80.0	77.5	75.0	72.5	69.9	67.2	64.6	61.9
90	94.3	92.3	90.2	88.0	85.7	83.4	80.9	78.5	75.9	73.3	70.7	68.1	65.4	62.7
91	95.5	93.4	91.3	89.1	86.8	84.4	81.9	79.4	76.9	74.2	71.6	68.9	66.2	63.5
92	96.6	94.6	92.4	90.1	87.8	85.4	82.9	80.4	77.8	75.1	72.5	69.7	67.0	64.2
93	97.8	95.7	93.5	91.2	88.9	86.4	83.9	81.3	78.7	76.0	73.3	70.6	67.8	65.0
94	98.9	96.8	94.6	92.3	89.9	87.4	84.9	82.3	79.6	76.9	74.2	71.4	68.6	65.8
95	100.1	97.9	95.7	93.4	91.0	88.5	85.9	83.3	80.6	77.8	75.1	72.2	69.4	66.5
96	101.3	99.1	96.8	94.4	92.0	89.5	86.9	84.2	81.5	78.7	75.9	73.1	70.2	67.3
97	102.4	100.2	97.9	95.5	93.1	90.5	87.9	85.2	82.4	79.6	76.8	73.9	71.0	68.1
98	103.6	101.4	99.0	96.6	94.1	91.5	88.9	86.2	83.4	80.5	77.7	74.7	71.8	68.8
99	104.7	102.5	100.1	97.7	95.2	92.6	89.9	87.1	84.3	81.5	78.5	75.6	72.6	69.6
100	105.9	103.6	101.3	98.8	96.2	93.6	90.9	88.1	85.3	82.4	79.4	76.4	73.4	70.4
101	107.1	104.8	102.4	99.9	97.3	94.6	91.9	89.1	86.2	83.3	80.3	77.3	74.2	71.2
102	108.2	105.9	103.5	101.0	98.4	95.7	92.9	90.0	87.1	84.2	81.2	78.1	75.0	71.9
103	109.4	107.1	104.6	102.1	99.4	96.7	93.9	91.0	88.1	85.1	82.0	79.0	75.8	72.7
104	110.6	108.2	105.7	103.1	100.5	97.7	94.9	92.0	89.0	86.0	82.9	79.8	76.6	73.5
105	111.7	109.3	106.8	104.2	101.5	98.8	95.9	93.0	90.0	86.9	83.8	80.6	77.5	74.3
106	112.9	110.5	108.0	105.3	102.6	99.8	96.9	93.9	90.9	87.8	84.7	81.5	78.3	75.0
107	114.1	111.6	109.1	106.4	103.7	100.8	97.9	94.9	91.8	88.7	85.5	82.3	79.1	75.8
108	115.3	112.8	110.2	107.5	104.7	101.9	98.9	95.9	92.8	89.6	86.4	83.2	79.9	76.6
109	116.4	113.9	111.3	108.6	105.8	102.9	99.9	96.9	93.7	90.5	87.3	84.0	80.7	77.4
110	117.6	115.1	112.4	109.7	106.9	103.9	100.9	97.8	94.7	91.5	88.2	84.9	81.5	78.2

TABLE XXV

CAUCASIAN AND ORIENTAL BOYS, LEAN BODY WEIGHT

Wrist: 17.0 cm

Weight (kg)	Knee (cm) 30	31	32	33	34	35	36	37	38	39	40	41	42	43
40	38.8	37.9	37.1	36.2	35.2	34.3	33.3	32.2	31.2	30.1	29.1	28.0	26.9	25.8
41	39.8	39.0	38.1	37.1	36.2	35.2	34.2	33.1	32.1	31.0	29.9	28.7	27.6	26.5
42	40.9	40.0	39.1	38.1	37.2	36.1	35.1	34.0	32.9	31.8	30.7	29.5	28.3	27.2
43	42.0	41.1	40.1	39.1	38.1	37.1	36.0	34.9	33.8	32.6	31.5	30.3	29.1	27.9
44	43.0	42.1	41.1	40.1	39.1	38.0	36.9	35.8	34.6	33.5	32.3	31.1	29.8	28.6
45	44.1	43.2	42.2	41.2	40.1	39.0	37.9	36.7	35.5	34.3	33.1	31.8	30.6	29.3
46	45.2	44.2	43.2	42.2	41.1	39.9	38.8	37.6	36.4	35.1	33.9	32.6	31.3	30.0
47	46.3	45.3	44.2	43.2	42.0	40.9	39.7	38.5	37.3	36.0	34.7	33.4	32.1	30.8
48	47.4	46.3	45.3	44.2	43.0	41.9	40.6	39.4	38.1	36.8	35.5	34.2	32.8	31.5
49	48.4	47.4	46.3	45.2	44.0	42.8	41.6	40.3	39.0	37.7	36.3	35.0	33.6	32.2
50	49.5	48.5	47.4	46.2	45.0	43.8	42.5	41.2	39.9	38.5	37.1	35.7	34.3	32.9
51	50.6	49.5	48.4	47.2	46.0	44.7	43.4	42.1	40.8	39.4	38.0	36.5	35.1	33.6
52	51.7	50.6	49.4	48.2	47.0	45.7	44.4	43.0	41.6	40.2	38.8	37.3	35.8	34.4
53	52.8	51.7	50.5	49.3	48.0	46.7	45.3	43.9	42.5	41.1	39.6	38.1	36.6	35.1
54	53.9	52.7	51.5	50.3	49.0	47.6	46.3	44.8	43.4	41.9	40.4	38.9	37.4	35.8
55	55.0	53.8	52.6	51.3	50.0	48.6	47.2	45.8	44.3	42.8	41.2	39.7	38.1	36.6
56	56.1	54.9	53.6	52.3	51.0	49.6	48.1	46.7	45.2	43.6	42.1	40.5	38.9	37.3
57	57.2	56.0	54.7	53.4	52.0	50.6	49.1	47.6	46.1	44.5	42.9	41.3	39.7	38.0
58	58.3	57.1	55.8	54.4	53.0	51.5	50.0	48.5	46.9	45.3	43.7	42.1	40.4	38.8
59	59.4	58.1	56.8	55.4	54.0	52.5	51.0	49.4	47.8	46.2	44.6	42.9	41.2	39.5
60	60.5	59.2	57.9	56.5	55.0	53.5	51.9	50.4	48.7	47.1	45.4	43.7	42.0	40.2
61	61.6	60.3	58.9	57.5	56.0	54.5	52.9	51.3	49.6	47.9	46.2	44.5	42.7	41.0
62	62.7	61.4	60.0	58.5	57.0	55.5	53.8	52.2	50.5	48.8	47.0	45.3	43.5	41.7
63	63.9	62.5	61.1	59.6	58.0	56.4	54.8	53.1	51.4	49.7	47.9	46.1	44.3	42.4
64	65.0	63.6	62.1	60.6	59.0	57.4	55.8	54.1	52.3	50.5	48.7	46.9	45.0	43.2
65	66.1	64.7	63.2	61.7	60.1	58.4	56.7	55.0	53.2	51.4	49.6	47.7	45.8	43.9
66	67.2	65.8	64.3	62.7	61.1	59.4	57.7	55.9	54.1	52.3	50.4	48.5	46.6	44.7
67	68.3	66.9	65.3	63.7	62.1	60.4	58.6	56.8	55.0	53.1	51.2	49.3	47.4	45.4
68	69.5	68.0	66.4	64.8	63.1	61.4	59.6	57.8	55.9	54.0	52.1	50.1	48.1	46.2
69	70.6	69.1	67.5	65.8	64.1	62.4	60.6	58.7	56.8	54.9	52.9	50.9	48.9	46.9
70	71.7	70.2	68.6	66.9	65.2	63.4	61.5	59.7	57.7	55.8	53.8	51.7	49.7	47.7
71	72.8	71.3	69.6	67.9	66.2	64.4	62.5	60.6	58.6	56.6	54.6	52.6	50.5	48.4
72	74.0	72.4	70.7	69.0	67.2	65.4	63.5	61.5	59.5	57.5	55.5	53.4	51.3	49.2
73	75.1	73.5	71.8	70.0	68.2	66.4	64.4	62.5	60.4	58.4	56.3	54.2	52.1	49.9
74	76.2	74.6	72.9	71.1	69.3	67.4	65.4	63.4	61.4	59.3	57.2	55.0	52.8	50.7
75	77.4	75.7	74.0	72.2	70.3	68.4	66.4	64.4	62.3	60.2	58.0	55.8	53.6	51.4
76	78.5	76.8	75.0	73.2	71.3	69.4	67.4	65.3	63.2	61.0	58.9	56.6	54.4	52.2
77	79.6	77.9	76.1	74.3	72.4	70.4	68.3	66.2	64.1	61.9	59.7	57.5	55.2	52.9
78	80.8	79.0	77.2	75.3	73.4	71.4	69.3	67.2	65.0	62.8	60.6	58.3	56.0	53.7
79	81.9	80.1	78.3	76.4	74.4	72.4	70.3	68.1	65.9	63.7	61.4	59.1	56.8	54.4
80	83.0	81.3	79.4	77.5	75.5	73.4	71.3	69.1	66.9	64.6	62.3	59.9	57.6	55.2
81	84.2	82.4	80.5	78.5	76.5	74.4	72.2	70.0	67.8	65.5	63.1	60.8	58.4	55.9
82	85.3	83.5	81.6	79.6	77.5	75.4	73.2	71.0	68.7	66.4	64.0	61.6	59.2	56.7
83	86.5	84.6	82.7	80.7	78.6	76.4	74.2	71.9	69.6	67.2	64.8	62.4	59.9	57.5
84	87.6	85.7	83.8	81.7	79.6	77.4	75.2	72.9	70.5	68.1	65.7	63.2	60.7	58.2
85	88.8	86.9	84.9	82.8	80.7	78.5	76.2	73.8	71.5	69.0	66.6	64.1	61.5	59.0
86	89.9	88.0	86.0	83.9	81.7	79.5	77.2	74.8	72.4	69.9	67.4	64.9	62.3	59.8
87	91.1	89.1	87.1	84.9	82.8	80.5	78.2	75.8	73.3	70.8	68.3	65.7	63.1	60.5
88	92.2	90.2	88.2	86.0	83.8	81.5	79.1	76.7	74.2	71.7	69.1	66.5	63.9	61.3
89	93.4	91.4	89.3	87.1	84.8	82.5	80.1	77.7	75.2	72.6	70.0	67.4	64.7	62.1
90	94.5	92.5	90.4	88.2	85.9	83.5	81.1	78.6	76.1	73.5	70.9	68.2	65.5	62.8
91	95.7	93.6	91.5	89.3	86.9	84.6	82.1	79.6	77.0	74.4	71.7	69.0	66.3	63.6
92	96.8	94.8	92.6	90.3	88.0	85.6	83.1	80.6	78.0	75.3	72.6	69.9	67.1	64.4
93	98.0	95.9	93.7	91.4	89.0	86.6	84.1	81.5	78.9	76.2	73.5	70.7	67.9	65.1
94	99.2	97.0	94.8	92.5	90.1	87.6	85.1	82.5	79.8	77.1	74.3	71.6	68.7	65.9
95	100.3	98.2	95.9	93.6	91.2	88.7	86.1	83.5	80.8	78.0	75.2	72.4	69.5	66.7
96	101.5	99.3	97.0	94.7	92.2	89.7	87.1	84.4	81.7	78.9	76.1	73.2	70.3	67.4
97	102.6	100.4	98.1	95.7	93.3	90.7	88.1	85.4	82.6	79.8	77.0	74.1	71.2	68.2
98	103.8	101.6	99.2	96.8	94.3	91.7	89.1	86.4	83.6	80.7	77.8	74.9	72.0	69.0
99	105.0	102.7	100.4	97.9	95.4	92.8	90.1	87.3	84.5	81.6	78.7	75.8	72.8	69.8
100	106.1	103.9	101.5	99.0	96.4	93.8	91.1	88.3	85.4	82.5	79.6	76.6	73.6	70.5
101	107.3	105.0	102.6	100.1	97.5	94.8	92.1	89.3	86.4	83.4	80.5	77.4	74.4	71.3
102	108.5	106.1	103.7	101.2	98.6	95.9	93.1	90.2	87.3	84.4	81.3	78.3	75.2	72.1
103	109.6	107.3	104.8	102.3	99.6	96.9	94.1	91.2	88.3	85.3	82.2	79.1	76.0	72.9
104	110.8	108.4	105.9	103.4	100.7	97.9	95.1	92.2	89.2	86.2	83.1	80.0	76.8	73.6
105	112.0	109.6	107.1	104.5	101.8	99.0	96.1	93.2	90.1	87.1	84.0	80.8	77.6	74.4
106	113.2	110.7	108.2	105.6	102.8	100.0	97.1	94.1	91.1	88.0	84.8	81.7	78.4	75.2
107	114.3	111.9	109.3	106.6	103.9	101.0	98.1	95.1	92.0	88.9	85.7	82.5	79.3	76.0
108	115.5	113.0	110.4	107.7	105.0	102.1	99.1	96.1	93.0	89.8	86.6	83.4	80.1	76.8
109	116.7	114.2	111.6	108.8	106.0	103.1	100.1	97.1	93.9	90.7	87.5	84.2	80.9	77.5
110	117.9	115.3	112.7	109.9	107.1	104.2	101.1	98.0	94.9	91.7	88.4	85.1	81.7	78.3

TABLE XXVI

CAUCASIAN AND ORIENTAL BOYS, LEAN BODY WEIGHT

Wrist: 17.5 cm

Weight (kg)	30	31	32	33	34	35	Knee (cm) 36	37	38	39	40	41	42	43
51	50.7	49.6	48.5	47.3	46.1	44.8	43.5	42.2	40.8	39.5	38.0	36.6	35.2	33.7
52	51.8	50.7	49.6	48.4	47.1	45.8	44.5	43.1	41.7	40.3	38.9	37.4	35.9	34.4
53	52.9	51.8	50.6	49.4	48.1	46.8	45.4	44.0	42.6	41.2	39.7	38.2	36.7	35.2
54	54.0	52.9	51.7	50.4	49.1	47.8	46.4	44.9	43.5	42.0	40.5	39.0	37.5	35.9
55	55.1	53.9	52.7	51.4	50.1	48.7	47.3	45.9	44.4	42.9	41.3	39.8	38.2	36.6
56	56.2	55.0	53.8	52.5	51.1	49.7	48.3	46.8	45.3	43.7	42.2	40.6	39.0	37.4
57	57.3	56.1	54.8	53.5	52.1	50.7	49.2	47.7	46.2	44.6	43.0	41.4	39.7	38.1
58	58.4	57.2	55.9	54.5	53.1	51.7	50.2	48.6	47.0	45.4	43.8	42.2	40.5	38.8
59	59.6	58.3	56.9	55.6	54.1	52.6	51.1	49.5	47.9	46.3	44.7	43.0	41.3	39.6
60	60.7	59.4	58.0	56.6	55.1	53.6	52.1	50.5	48.8	47.2	45.5	43.8	42.1	40.3
61	61.8	60.5	59.1	57.6	56.1	54.6	53.0	51.4	49.7	48.0	46.3	44.6	42.8	41.1
62	62.9	61.5	60.1	58.7	57.1	55.6	54.0	52.3	50.6	48.9	47.2	45.4	43.6	41.8
63	64.0	62.6	61.2	59.7	58.2	56.6	54.9	53.2	51.5	49.8	48.0	46.2	44.4	42.5
64	65.1	63.7	62.3	60.8	59.2	57.6	55.9	54.2	52.4	50.6	48.8	47.0	45.1	43.3
65	66.2	64.8	63.3	61.8	60.2	58.5	56.8	55.1	53.3	51.5	49.7	47.8	45.9	44.0
66	67.4	65.9	64.4	62.8	61.2	59.5	57.8	56.0	54.2	52.4	50.5	48.6	46.7	44.8
67	68.5	67.0	65.5	63.9	62.2	60.5	58.8	57.0	55.1	53.3	51.4	49.4	47.5	45.5
68	69.6	68.1	66.6	64.9	63.3	61.5	59.7	57.9	56.0	54.1	52.2	50.2	48.3	46.3
69	70.7	69.2	67.6	66.0	64.3	62.5	60.7	58.8	56.9	55.0	53.0	51.1	49.0	47.0
70	71.9	70.3	68.7	67.0	65.3	63.5	61.7	59.8	57.9	55.9	53.9	51.9	49.8	47.8
71	73.0	71.4	69.8	68.1	66.3	64.5	62.6	60.7	58.8	56.8	54.7	52.7	50.6	48.5
72	74.1	72.5	70.9	69.1	67.4	65.5	63.6	61.7	59.7	57.6	55.6	53.5	51.4	49.3
73	75.3	73.6	72.0	70.2	68.4	66.5	64.6	62.6	60.6	58.5	56.4	54.3	52.2	50.0
74	76.4	74.8	73.0	71.3	69.4	67.5	65.6	63.6	61.5	59.4	57.3	55.1	53.0	50.8
75	77.5	75.9	74.1	72.3	70.5	68.5	66.5	64.5	62.4	60.3	58.1	56.0	53.7	51.5
76	78.7	77.0	75.2	73.4	71.5	69.5	67.5	65.4	63.3	61.2	59.0	56.8	54.5	52.3
77	79.8	78.1	76.3	74.4	72.5	70.5	68.5	66.4	64.2	62.1	59.8	57.6	55.3	53.0
78	80.9	79.2	77.4	75.5	73.6	71.5	69.5	67.3	65.2	62.9	60.7	58.4	56.1	53.8
79	82.1	80.3	78.5	76.6	74.6	72.6	70.4	68.3	66.1	63.8	61.6	59.2	56.9	54.6
80	83.2	81.4	79.6	77.6	75.6	73.6	71.4	69.2	67.0	64.7	62.4	60.1	57.7	55.3
81	84.4	82.6	80.7	78.7	76.7	74.6	72.4	70.2	67.9	65.6	63.3	60.9	58.5	56.1
82	85.5	83.7	81.8	79.8	77.7	75.6	73.4	71.1	68.8	66.5	64.1	61.7	59.3	56.8
83	86.7	84.8	82.9	80.8	78.8	76.6	74.4	72.1	69.8	67.4	65.0	62.5	60.1	57.6
84	87.8	85.9	84.0	81.9	79.8	77.6	75.4	73.1	70.7	68.3	65.9	63.4	60.9	58.4
85	89.0	87.1	85.1	83.0	80.8	78.6	76.4	74.0	71.6	69.2	66.7	64.2	61.7	59.1
86	90.1	88.2	86.2	84.1	81.9	79.6	77.3	75.0	72.6	70.1	67.6	65.0	62.5	59.9
87	91.3	89.3	87.3	85.1	82.9	80.7	78.3	75.9	73.5	71.0	68.4	65.9	63.3	60.7
88	92.4	90.4	88.4	86.2	84.0	81.7	79.3	76.9	74.4	71.9	69.3	66.7	64.1	61.4
89	93.6	91.6	89.5	87.3	85.0	82.7	80.3	77.9	75.3	72.8	70.2	67.5	64.9	62.2
90	94.7	92.7	90.6	88.4	86.1	83.7	81.3	78.8	76.3	73.7	71.0	68.4	65.7	63.0
91	95.9	93.8	91.7	89.5	87.1	84.8	82.3	79.8	77.2	74.6	71.9	69.2	66.5	63.7
92	97.1	95.0	92.8	90.5	88.2	85.8	83.3	80.7	78.1	75.5	72.8	70.0	67.3	64.5
93	98.2	96.1	93.9	91.6	89.3	86.8	84.3	81.7	79.1	76.4	73.6	70.9	68.1	65.3
94	99.4	97.2	95.0	92.7	90.3	87.8	85.3	82.7	80.0	77.3	74.5	71.7	68.9	66.0
95	100.5	98.4	96.1	93.8	91.4	88.9	86.3	83.6	80.9	78.2	75.4	72.6	69.7	66.8
96	101.7	99.5	97.2	94.9	92.4	89.9	87.3	84.6	81.9	79.1	76.3	73.4	70.5	67.6
97	102.9	100.7	98.4	96.0	93.5	90.9	88.3	85.6	82.8	80.0	77.1	74.2	71.3	68.4
98	104.0	101.8	99.5	97.1	94.5	91.9	89.3	86.5	83.8	80.9	78.0	75.1	72.1	69.1
99	105.2	102.9	100.6	98.1	95.6	93.0	90.3	87.5	84.7	81.8	78.9	75.9	72.9	69.9
100	106.4	104.1	101.7	99.2	96.7	94.0	91.3	88.5	85.6	82.7	79.8	76.8	73.7	70.7
101	107.5	105.2	102.8	100.3	97.7	95.0	92.3	89.5	86.6	83.6	80.6	77.6	74.6	71.5
102	108.7	106.4	103.9	101.4	98.8	96.1	93.3	90.4	87.5	84.5	81.5	78.5	75.4	72.3
103	109.9	107.5	105.1	102.5	99.9	97.1	94.3	91.4	88.5	85.5	82.4	79.3	76.2	73.0
104	111.1	108.7	106.2	103.6	100.9	98.2	95.3	92.4	89.4	86.4	83.3	80.1	77.0	73.8
105	112.2	109.8	107.3	104.7	102.0	99.2	96.3	93.4	90.4	87.3	84.2	81.0	77.8	74.6
106	113.4	111.0	108.4	105.8	103.1	100.2	97.3	94.3	91.3	88.2	85.0	81.8	78.6	75.4
107	114.6	112.1	109.6	106.9	104.1	101.3	98.3	95.3	92.2	89.1	85.9	82.7	79.4	76.2
108	115.8	113.3	110.7	108.0	105.2	102.3	99.3	96.3	93.2	90.0	86.8	83.5	80.3	76.9
109	116.9	114.4	111.8	109.1	106.3	103.4	100.4	97.3	94.1	90.9	87.7	84.4	81.1	77.7
110	118.1	115.6	112.9	110.2	107.3	104.4	101.4	98.3	95.1	91.9	88.6	85.2	81.9	78.5

TABLE XXVII

CAUCASIAN AND ORIENTAL BOYS, LEAN BODY WEIGHT

Wrist: 18.0 cm

Weight (kg)	30	31	32	33	34	35	Knee (cm) 36	37	38	39	40	41	42	43
51	50.9	49.8	48.6	47.4	46.2	45.0	43.6	42.3	40.9	39.6	38.1	36.7	35.3	33.8
52	52.0	50.8	49.7	48.5	47.2	45.9	44.6	43.2	41.8	40.4	39.0	37.5	36.0	34.5
53	53.1	51.9	50.7	49.5	48.2	46.9	45.5	44.1	42.7	41.3	39.8	38.3	36.8	35.3
54	54.2	53.0	51.8	50.5	49.2	47.9	46.5	45.1	43.6	42.1	40.6	39.1	37.5	36.0
55	55.3	54.1	52.8	51.6	50.2	48.8	47.4	46.0	44.5	43.0	41.4	39.9	38.3	36.7
56	56.4	55.2	53.9	52.6	51.2	49.8	48.4	46.9	45.4	43.8	42.3	40.7	39.1	37.5
57	57.5	56.2	55.0	53.6	52.2	50.8	49.3	47.8	46.3	44.7	43.1	41.5	39.8	38.2
58	58.6	57.3	56.0	54.7	53.2	51.8	50.3	48.7	47.2	45.6	43.9	42.3	40.6	38.9
59	59.7	58.4	57.1	55.7	54.2	52.8	51.2	49.7	48.1	46.4	44.8	43.1	41.4	39.7
60	60.8	59.5	58.1	56.7	55.3	53.7	52.2	50.6	49.0	47.3	45.6	43.9	42.2	40.4
61	61.9	60.6	59.2	57.8	56.3	54.7	53.1	51.5	49.9	48.2	46.4	44.7	42.9	41.2
62	63.0	61.7	60.3	58.8	57.3	55.7	54.1	52.4	50.8	49.0	47.3	45.5	43.7	41.9
63	64.2	62.8	61.3	59.9	58.3	56.7	55.1	53.4	51.7	49.9	48.1	46.3	44.5	42.6
64	65.3	63.9	62.4	60.9	59.3	57.7	56.0	54.3	52.6	50.8	49.0	47.1	45.3	43.4
65	66.4	65.0	63.5	61.9	60.3	58.7	57.0	55.2	53.5	51.6	49.8	47.9	46.0	44.1
66	67.5	66.1	64.6	63.0	61.4	59.7	58.0	56.2	54.4	52.5	50.6	48.7	46.8	44.9
67	68.7	67.2	65.6	64.0	62.4	60.7	58.9	57.1	55.3	53.4	51.5	49.5	47.6	45.6
68	69.8	68.3	66.7	65.1	63.4	61.7	59.9	58.1	56.2	54.3	52.3	50.4	48.4	46.4
69	70.9	69.4	67.8	66.1	64.4	62.7	60.9	59.0	57.1	55.1	53.2	51.2	49.2	47.1
70	72.0	70.5	68.9	67.2	65.5	63.7	61.8	59.9	58.0	56.0	54.0	52.0	49.9	47.9
71	73.2	71.6	70.0	68.3	66.5	64.7	62.8	60.9	58.9	56.9	54.9	52.8	50.7	48.6
72	74.3	72.7	71.0	69.3	67.5	65.7	63.8	61.8	59.8	57.8	55.7	53.6	51.5	49.4
73	75.4	73.8	72.1	70.4	68.6	66.7	64.7	62.8	60.7	58.7	56.6	54.4	52.3	50.1
74	76.6	74.9	73.2	71.4	69.6	67.7	65.7	63.7	61.7	59.6	57.4	55.3	53.1	50.9
75	77.7	76.1	74.3	72.5	70.6	68.7	66.7	64.7	62.6	60.4	58.3	56.1	53.9	51.7
76	78.9	77.2	75.4	73.6	71.7	69.7	67.7	65.6	63.5	61.3	59.1	56.9	54.7	52.4
77	80.0	78.3	76.5	74.6	72.7	70.7	68.7	66.6	64.4	62.2	60.0	57.7	55.5	53.2
78	81.1	79.4	77.6	75.7	73.7	71.7	69.6	67.5	65.3	63.1	60.8	58.6	56.3	53.9
79	82.3	80.5	78.7	76.8	74.8	72.7	70.6	68.5	66.2	64.0	61.7	59.4	57.0	54.7
80	83.4	81.6	79.8	77.8	75.8	73.7	71.6	69.4	67.2	64.9	62.6	60.2	57.8	55.5
81	84.6	82.8	80.9	78.9	76.9	74.8	72.6	70.4	68.1	65.8	63.4	61.0	58.6	56.2
82	85.7	83.9	82.0	80.0	77.9	75.8	73.6	71.3	69.0	66.7	64.3	61.9	59.4	57.0
83	86.9	85.0	83.1	81.0	78.9	76.8	74.6	72.3	69.9	67.6	65.1	62.7	60.2	57.7
84	88.0	86.1	84.2	82.1	80.0	77.8	75.5	73.2	70.9	68.5	66.0	63.5	61.0	58.5
85	89.2	87.3	85.3	83.2	81.0	78.8	76.5	74.2	71.8	69.4	66.9	64.4	61.8	59.3
86	90.3	88.4	86.4	84.3	82.1	79.8	77.5	75.2	72.7	70.3	67.7	65.2	62.6	60.0
87	91.5	89.5	87.5	85.3	83.1	80.9	78.5	76.1	73.7	71.2	68.6	66.0	63.4	60.8
88	92.7	90.7	88.6	86.4	84.2	81.9	79.5	77.1	74.6	72.1	69.5	66.9	64.2	61.6
89	93.8	91.8	89.7	87.5	85.2	82.9	80.5	78.0	75.5	73.0	70.3	67.7	65.0	62.3
90	95.0	92.9	90.8	88.6	86.3	83.9	81.5	79.0	76.5	73.9	71.2	68.5	65.8	63.1
91	96.1	94.1	91.9	89.7	87.4	85.0	82.5	80.0	77.4	74.8	72.1	69.4	66.6	63.9
92	97.3	95.2	93.0	90.8	88.4	86.0	83.5	80.9	78.3	75.7	73.0	70.2	67.4	64.7
93	98.5	96.3	94.1	91.8	89.5	87.0	84.5	81.9	79.3	76.6	73.8	71.1	68.3	65.4
94	99.6	97.5	95.2	92.9	90.5	88.0	85.5	82.9	80.2	77.5	74.7	71.9	69.1	66.2
95	100.8	98.6	96.4	94.0	91.6	89.1	86.5	83.8	81.1	78.4	75.6	72.7	69.9	67.0
96	102.0	99.8	97.5	95.1	92.6	90.1	87.5	84.8	82.1	79.3	76.4	73.6	70.7	67.8
97	103.1	100.9	98.6	96.2	93.7	91.1	88.5	85.8	83.0	80.2	77.3	74.4	71.5	68.5
98	104.3	102.1	99.7	97.3	94.8	92.2	89.5	86.8	84.0	81.1	78.2	75.3	72.3	69.3
99	105.5	103.2	100.8	98.4	95.8	93.2	90.5	87.7	84.9	82.0	79.1	76.1	73.1	70.1
100	106.6	104.3	102.0	99.5	96.9	94.2	91.5	88.7	85.8	82.9	80.0	77.0	73.9	70.9
101	107.8	105.5	103.1	100.6	98.0	95.3	92.5	89.7	86.8	83.8	80.8	77.8	74.7	71.6
102	109.0	106.6	104.2	101.7	99.0	96.3	93.5	90.7	87.7	84.7	81.7	78.6	75.5	72.4
103	110.2	107.8	105.3	102.8	100.1	97.4	94.5	91.6	88.7	85.7	82.6	79.5	76.4	73.2
104	111.3	108.9	106.4	103.9	101.2	98.4	95.5	92.6	89.6	86.6	83.5	80.3	77.2	74.0
105	112.5	110.1	107.6	105.0	102.2	99.4	96.6	93.6	90.6	87.5	84.4	81.2	78.0	74.8
106	113.7	111.2	108.7	106.1	103.3	100.5	97.6	94.6	91.5	88.4	85.2	82.0	78.8	75.6
107	114.9	112.4	109.8	107.2	104.4	101.5	98.6	95.6	92.5	89.3	86.1	82.9	79.6	76.3
108	116.1	113.6	111.0	108.3	105.5	102.6	99.6	96.5	93.4	90.2	87.0	83.7	80.4	77.1
109	117.2	114.7	112.1	109.4	106.5	103.6	100.6	97.5	94.4	91.2	87.9	84.6	81.3	77.9
110	118.4	115.9	113.2	110.5	107.6	104.7	101.6	98.5	95.3	92.1	88.8	85.5	82.1	78.7

TABLE XXVIII

CAUCASIAN AND ORIENTAL BOYS, LEAN BODY WEIGHT

Wrist: 18.5 cm

Weight (kg)	30	31	32	33	34	35	Knee (cm) 36	37	38	39	40	41	42	43
72	74.5	72.9	71.2	69.5	67.7	65.8	63.9	62.0	60.0	57.9	55.9	53.8	51.6	49.5
73	75.6	74.0	72.3	70.6	68.7	66.8	64.9	62.9	60.9	58.8	56.7	54.6	52.4	50.3
74	76.8	75.1	73.4	71.6	69.8	67.9	65.9	63.9	61.8	59.7	57.6	55.4	53.2	51.0
75	77.9	76.2	74.5	72.7	70.8	68.9	66.9	64.8	62.7	60.6	58.4	56.2	54.0	51.8
76	79.1	77.4	75.6	73.8	71.8	69.9	67.8	65.8	63.6	61.5	59.3	57.1	54.8	52.5
77	80.2	78.5	76.7	74.8	72.9	70.9	68.8	66.7	64.6	62.4	60.1	57.9	55.6	53.3
78	81.4	79.6	77.8	75.9	73.9	71.9	69.8	67.7	65.5	63.3	61.0	58.7	56.4	54.1
79	82.5	80.7	78.9	77.0	75.0	72.9	70.8	68.6	66.4	64.2	61.9	59.5	57.2	54.8
80	83.6	81.9	80.0	78.0	76.0	73.9	71.8	69.6	67.3	65.0	62.7	60.4	58.0	55.6
81	84.8	83.0	81.1	79.1	77.1	74.9	72.8	70.5	68.3	65.9	63.6	61.2	58.8	56.4
82	86.0	84.1	82.2	80.2	78.1	76.0	73.8	71.5	69.2	66.8	64.4	62.0	59.6	57.1
83	87.1	85.2	83.3	81.3	79.2	77.0	74.8	72.5	70.1	67.7	65.3	62.9	60.4	57.9
84	88.3	86.4	84.4	82.3	80.2	78.0	75.7	73.4	71.1	68.6	66.2	63.7	61.2	58.7
85	89.4	87.5	85.5	83.4	81.3	79.0	76.7	74.4	72.0	69.5	67.0	64.5	62.0	59.4
86	90.6	88.6	86.6	84.5	82.3	80.0	77.7	75.3	72.9	70.4	67.9	65.4	62.8	60.2
87	91.7	89.8	87.7	85.6	83.4	81.1	78.7	76.3	73.8	71.3	68.8	66.2	63.6	61.0
88	92.9	90.9	88.8	86.7	84.4	82.1	79.7	77.3	74.8	72.2	69.7	67.0	64.4	61.7
89	94.1	92.0	89.9	87.7	85.5	83.1	80.7	78.2	75.7	73.1	70.5	67.9	65.2	62.5
90	95.2	93.2	91.0	88.8	86.5	84.2	81.7	79.2	76.6	74.0	71.4	68.7	66.0	63.3
91	96.4	94.3	92.1	89.9	87.6	85.2	82.7	80.2	77.6	74.9	72.3	69.6	66.8	64.1
92	97.5	95.4	93.3	91.0	88.6	86.2	83.7	81.1	78.5	75.9	73.1	70.4	67.6	64.8
93	98.7	96.6	94.4	92.1	89.7	87.2	84.7	82.1	79.5	76.8	74.0	71.2	68.4	65.6
94	99.9	97.7	95.5	93.2	90.8	88.3	85.7	83.1	80.4	77.7	74.9	72.1	69.2	66.4
95	101.0	98.9	96.6	94.3	91.8	89.3	86.7	84.1	81.3	78.6	75.8	72.9	70.0	67.2
96	102.2	100.0	97.7	95.3	92.9	90.3	87.7	85.0	82.3	79.5	76.6	73.8	70.9	67.9
97	103.4	101.2	98.8	96.4	93.9	91.4	88.7	86.0	83.2	80.4	77.5	74.6	71.7	68.7
98	104.6	102.3	100.0	97.5	95.0	92.4	89.7	87.0	84.2	81.3	78.4	75.5	72.5	69.5
99	105.7	103.5	101.1	98.6	96.1	93.4	90.7	88.0	85.1	82.2	79.3	76.3	73.3	70.3
100	106.9	104.6	102.2	99.7	97.1	94.5	91.7	88.9	86.1	83.1	80.2	77.2	74.1	71.1
101	108.1	105.8	103.3	100.8	98.2	95.5	92.8	89.9	87.0	84.1	81.0	78.0	74.9	71.8
102	109.3	106.9	104.5	101.9	99.3	96.6	93.8	90.9	88.0	85.0	81.9	78.8	75.7	72.6
103	110.4	108.1	105.6	103.0	100.4	97.6	94.8	91.9	88.9	85.9	82.8	79.7	76.6	73.4
104	111.6	109.2	106.7	104.1	101.4	98.6	95.8	92.9	89.9	86.8	83.7	80.6	77.4	74.2
105	112.8	110.4	107.8	105.2	102.5	99.7	96.8	93.8	90.8	87.7	84.6	81.4	78.2	75.0
106	114.0	111.5	109.0	106.3	103.6	100.7	97.8	94.8	91.8	88.6	85.5	82.3	79.0	75.8
107	115.2	112.7	110.1	107.4	104.6	101.8	98.8	95.8	92.7	89.6	86.4	83.1	79.8	76.5
108	116.3	113.8	111.2	108.5	105.7	102.8	99.8	96.8	93.7	90.5	87.2	84.0	80.7	77.3
109	117.5	115.0	112.4	109.6	106.8	103.9	100.9	97.8	94.6	91.4	88.1	84.8	81.5	78.1
110	118.7	116.2	113.5	110.7	107.9	104.9	101.9	98.8	95.6	92.3	89.0	85.7	82.3	78.9

FORMS USED IN THE STUDY

Dear Student:

YOU HAVE BEEN CHOSEN.

"WHAT FOR?" you ask?

For the next step in the body measurement project.

WHAT *IS* THE NEXT STEP?—We'd like to study your eating habits. and measure your physical activity.

WHY?—We've already learned a lot about your muscle, fat, and bone from the measurements and profile. Now we'd like to know more about some of the habits that may have an effect on the amount and location of muscle and fat in your body.

ANYTHING ELSE?—You may be asked to take part in some other simple tests, all having to do with body composition.

WHERE?—At the School of Public Health, University of California at Berkeley.

WHEN?—One week, late in June 1963, at the end of the school year. We'll want to see you for about an hour each day, either morning or afternoon.

GUARANTEE—Painless. Also, we'll send you a report of what we find out about you.

In a few weeks you'll get another letter with more information so you can talk it over with the folks at home. Meanwhile, keep the project in mind.

THE MEASURING TEAM

May 26, 1964

Dear Student:

The school year is practically over and we're all ready and waiting to work with you again on diaries of your food and activities. Of course we hope you're ready and willing to keep the diaries again, as you did last spring and summer (however, there will be no body measuring this summer). You'll remember that we talked about the difficulties of learning about what people really eat and do if they keep records for only one week out of a summer. So we asked you to keep a record during the school year to add to the first one. Once again we hope you'll continue to fill in the detailed picture of YOU by recording another week this summer.

The procedure is the same as last spring: record everything you do and everything you eat for seven days, and bring the records in for checking each day either at the Odd Fellows Hall or the School of Public Health. As usual, we'll have office hours from 8:00 A.M. to 5:00 P.M. If you're working and those hours don't fit, others can be arranged. Yes, you got the message: we *do* want *you*. Again there will be a small gift for those who complete this summer project.

Please talk it over with your family. Then fill out the enclosed sheet and return it in the envelope as soon as you can. We will tell you your exact appointment time and place as soon as we hear from you. If there are questions, please phone TH 5–6000, Extension 4188, and talk with Mrs. Lynne Ramsey or Mrs. Barbara Mitchell.

We hope to hear from you soon and see you again this summer.

THE MEASURING TEAM

University of California
Department of Public Health
Family Information

STUDENT: Name _____

Present address _____

Permanent address _____

_____

Social Security Number _____

PARENTS: Highest School Grade Completed (Please check)

Father		*Mother*
_____	6th grade	_____
_____	7th grade	_____
_____	8th grade	_____
_____	9th grade	_____
_____	10th grade	_____
_____	11th grade	_____
_____	12th grade	_____

_____ College, year 1 _____
_____ College, year 2 _____
_____ College, year 3 _____
_____ College, year 4 _____
_____ College, year 5 _____
_____ College, year 6 _____
_____ College, year 7+ _____

Employer: Father _____
        Mother _____
Job Title: Father _____
        Mother _____

	Father	Mother
Weight:	_____	_____
Height:	_____	_____

GRANDPARENTS:
(if living)

	Father	Mother
Mother's Parents:	Father	Mother
Weight:	_____	_____
Height:	_____	_____
Father's Parents:	Father	Mother
Weight:	_____	_____
Height:	_____	_____

INSTRUCTIONS FOR KEEPING DIARIES

As a scientist, it is most important that you keep your diary accurately each day. For this diary record we will consider that the day starts at 12:00 midnight and continues until the following midnight (24 hours). You will start your record tomorrow. If you happen to be up past midnight tonight, record anything you eat, drink, or do after that time on your diary form, and the time.

Recording Food

In recording the food you eat, you will notice that there is a column labeled *how it was prepared*. If it is something like a raw apple, we won't care how it was prepared. If, however, it should be something like a roast beef sandwich, we want to know if butter or mayonnaise, or both, were used on it. If it included lettuce, or cheese, or tomatoes, we want to know about that, too. If it is a mixed dish, such as stew, or a casserole of some sort, we would like a recipe, if possible. If this is not possible, do your best to describe what the dish contained.

Amounts of food in the *how much* column are often a little bit difficult to describe. (We have some food models which may help you to decide how much you ate—you may look at them if you like. We consider most of the models to be *one serving* of that kind of food.) We will ask you, however, to measure as many of the things you eat as you possibly can. To do this you will need a plastic ruler six inches long, a measuring cup (standard household measure), and measuring spoons. The ruler, measuring cup, and spoons should be kept clean.

MEAT: Measure your portion of meat by thickness, length, and width, with your ruler and record whether or not you ate the fat.

FISH: Measure with your ruler, and record what kind of fish it is.

SMALL VEGETABLES: Peas, green beans, or corn (not corn on the cob) should be measured in a measuring cup.

MASHED POTATOES, RICE, BREAKFAST CEREALS (either dry or cooked), AND SALADS: All should be measured in a measuring cup.

FLUIDS: Water, milk, juice, coffee, or tea should be measured in a measuring cup. Things like milk and orange juice that you might usually drink out of the same glass need not be measured each day. But you should measure how much the glass contains when filled to the usual level. To do this, fill the glass to the customary level with water and then empty the water into a standard household measuring cup, and see if the glass holds 1 cup, ¾ cup, or even 1¼ cups.

CREAM AND SUGAR ADDED TO COFFEE AND TEA: Measure the amount with your measuring spoons before you add them to your drink.

BOTTLED SOFT DRINKS: The number of ounces the bottle contains is printed on the label. Write down the number of ounces on the diary sheet.

COOKIES: Measure the diameter and thickness with your ruler.

CAKE: Measure height as well as length and width, and record type of frosting, if any.

PIE: Measure height as well as width at crust, and length.

APPLE OR ORANGE: Cut in half before eating and measure the diameter with your ruler.

JAMS, PEANUT BUTTER and other foods which you use in fairly small quantities: Measure these items with your measuring spoons.

SALAD DRESSING AND MAYONNAISE: Look at the jar to see which it is, and measure the amounts with your measuring spoons.

CANDY BARS: the *kind,* and either the weight printed on the wrapper, or the cost.

Recording Activity

Bathing, face washing, going to the bathroom, taking clothes off or putting them on, are all a part of dressing or undressing and may be called "dressing."

Count and record all steps that you walk *up* during each day.

If you are sitting or reading for an hour or two and get up once or twice to get something to eat or drink, please record the amount of time spent walking and standing. Also, it is necessary to record what you ate or drank, and at what time you ate or drank it.

It is as important for us to know at what *times* you eat and drink as it is to know *what* it was and *how much* of it you ate or drank.

We realize that keeping these records is a difficult thing to do. But by keeping them you are helping to increase scientific knowledge, and so it is very important to keep them accurately. We know you realize the importance of keeping them honestly and carefully, and will do everything that you can to make this study a success.

We do not want you to do anything special or eat anything special—we just want to know what you do and eat this week. Please do not refrain from eating something or doing something that you usually eat or do, and please do not do or eat anything that you would not ordinarily do or eat. We do not care what you do, but we must *know* what you do.

Name_____ Record Number_____

(First)   (Middle)   (Last)   Phone Number_____

Address_____

Diary for: Day_____ (Date)_____

Time Started	Time Stopped	What I Did	Duration SI VL L M S	What I Ate	How Much	How It Was Prepared
			(leave blank)			

SUMMARY SHEET FOR WEEK'S ACTIVITY RECORD AND PEDOMETER READINGS

Type of Activity	Very Light x 1	Light x 2	Moderate x 3	Strenuous x 4	Very Strenuous x 5	Sleeping	Total	Pedometer Reading Each Day
				Duration				
Day 1								
Day 2								
Day 3								
Day 4								
Day 5								
Day 6								
Day 7								
Total for Week								
Total in Hours & Tenths of Hours								
Total x Factor							Total Score	

September 1964

ANTHROPOMETRIC EVALUATION

☐ _____

Name_____

Address_____

Identification Code_____

Date of Examination_____

Date of Birth_____

Stature_____dm._____in.

Weight_____kg._____lbs.

Circumferences (cm.):

    Shoulder_____

    Chest_____

    Abdomen: Upper_____

             Lower_____

    Buttocks_____

    Thigh   R_____L_____

_____

_____

    Biceps R_____L_____

    Forearm R_____L_____

    Wrist R_____L_____

    Knee R_____L_____

    Calf   R_____L_____

    Ankle R_____L_____   Deltoid R_____L_____

_____

_____

Diameters (cm.):

    Chest_____   Bi Deltoid_____

    Bitrochanteric_____   Knees R_____L_____

    Wrist R_____L_____   Elbows R_____L_____

    Ankle R_____L_____

    Bi-iliac_____

    Biacromial_____

You realize that all the information we gather will be kept confidential, and that any report made either to parents or schools will not give your names.

INFORMATION FOR WATER DISPLACEMENT TEST

The water displacement test, or weighing under water as it may be called, is a method of finding out your body volume and therefore your body density.

The amount you weigh in air subtracted from the amount you weigh in water indicates the weight of water displaced by your body. This weight of water can easily be calculated to the equivalent volume of water. This represents the volume of your body. The density of your body is its weight divided by its volume. From this we can determine the approximate amount of fat, bone, and muscle, since bone is the most dense and fat the least dense of these three kinds of body tissue.

The tank that we use for underwater weighing is about four feet deep, so anyone can stand up in it easily. To do the weighing, we will ask you to get into the tank and sit on a little swing suspended from scales. When we are ready to do the weighing, we will ask you to lean over and put your head under water.

We will provide swim suits and swim caps for the girls. Boys are asked to bring their own swim trunks. Towels and dressing facilities will be available.

INFORMATION FOR POTASSIUM^{40} COUNTER

Perhaps you know that there are some radioisotopes of common elements that occur in nature. These have been useful for many things. One of the most interesting uses of this natural phenomenon is the measurement of carbon^{14} in archeological specimens to determine their age. This is called "carbon dating." The principle involved in carbon dating is really quite simple. Usually the carbon atom found in living matter has an atomic weight of 12 and is called carbon^{12}. There is, however, a little carbon^{14} (carbon with an atomic weight of 14) found in nature. This carbon^{14} is constantly being formed by cosmic rays hitting the earth. It is also constantly decaying and becoming carbon^{12} again, so that on the surface of the earth growing things are incorporating about the same proportion of carbon^{14} to carbon^{12} in their structure all the time. If a material is buried (as with archeological specimens) and no longer exposed to cosmic rays, the proportion of carbon^{14} to carbon^{12} gradually decreases. By measuring this proportion with very sensitive instruments, a scientist can determine approximately how old any carbon-containing material might be.

What we want to do is apply this principle to you.

The atomic weight of potassium is usually 39, but there is always a certain small proportion of potassium^{40} in nature formed by cosmic rays. Potassium is a chemical element found in the human body in the bones and muscles. There is very little potassium found in fat tissue. Thus if we measure the amount of potassium^{40} which is naturally in your body we can calculate the total amount of potassium in your body, and from that determine how much of your body is bone, muscle, and fat.

The process for measuring the potassium^{40} is fairly simple. You will be asked to sit quietly, alone in a room which will have in it some very sensitive instruments. These instruments will measure or really count the tiny particles given off by the naturally occurring potassium^{40} in your body. Of course you will have to be alone in the room, because everyone has potassium^{40} in his body, and anyone else in the room would affect the counting instruments as much as you would.

Please wash your hair thoroughly the night before being "counted," as there might be some tiny dust particles in your hair that would affect the delicate instruments.

Name:_____

QUESTIONNAIRE

This is *not* a test. It is a questionnaire designed to find out how *you* feel about these things. There are no right or wrong answers. For some questions, you may wish to check more than one answer.

1. Which meal do you like best?_____

   Why?_____

   _____

   _____

   _____

   _____

2. In your opinion which person in your family or among your friends has the best idea about good-tasting foods?_____

   _____

3. A. Do you think that you are

   _____ Quite a lot too thin?

   _____ A little bit too thin?

   _____ About right?

   _____ A little bit too fat?

   _____ Quite a lot too fat?

   B. Are you trying to do anything about your weight?

   _____ Yes

   _____ No

Name: _____

C. If your answer is "yes", please explain what you are trying to do._____

_____

_____

_____

_____

_____

4. How often are you hungry?

_____ All the time

_____ Most of the time

_____ Some of the time

_____ Hardly ever

_____ Never

Check on the line below the approximate time of the day when you are usually the most hungry:

Earlier 6 a.m. 9 a.m. 12 Noon 3 p.m. 6 p.m. 9 p.m. Later
than 6 a.m.   than 9 p.m.

5. What foods should be eaten every day for health?_____

_____

_____

_____

_____

_____

Name:_____

6. How much would you like to weigh?
   _____ 10 to 20 pounds more than you do now
   _____ 5 to 10 pounds more than you do now
   _____ 1 to 5 pounds more than you do now
   _____ Exactly the number of pounds you weigh now
   _____ 1 to 5 pounds less than you do now
   _____ 5 to 10 pounds less than you do now
   _____ 10 to 20 pounds less than you do now

7. If a person is fat, which of the following is most likely to be the reason?
   _____ It is natural for him to be fat.
   _____ He doesn't exercise enough.
   _____ He eats too much.
   _____ Other (explain) _____

   _____

8. A. How would you grade the healthfulness of what you eat?

   _____ Poor
   _____ Fair
   _____ Good
   _____ Excellent

   B. If you think it needs improving, how do you think it should be changed?_____

   _____

   _____

   _____

   _____

Name:_____

9. How would you describe yourself physically?

_____ Very inactive

_____ Inactive

_____ Average

_____ Active

_____ Very Active

10. A. Some people say teenagers don't eat the right foods. Do you agree with the people who say this?

_____ Yes

_____ No

B. Why do you agree or disagree?_____

_____

_____

_____

_____

_____

11. This is a question to find out how much you like or dislike certain activities. For each activity listed, draw a circle around the reply which tells how much you like or dislike it. Draw only one circle for each activity.

Example 1: If you have ever gone hiking and you dislike hiking a little, circle "Dislike a Little" after hiking, as shown below.

HIKING	Not Tried	Like Very Much	Like a Little	Neither Like Nor Dislike	Dislike a Little	Dislike Very Much

Name:_____

Example 2: If you have never tried hiking so you don't know whether you like or dislike it, circle "Not Tried" for that activity, as shown below.

HIKING	(Not Tried)	Like Very Much	Like a Little	Neither Like Nor Dislike	Dislike a Little	Dislike Very Much

START HERE:

LISTENING TO RADIO OR RECORDS	Not Tried	Like Very Much	Like a Little	Neither Like Nor Dislike	Dislike a Little	Dislike Very Much
DANCING	Not Tried	Like Very Much	Like a Little	Neither Like Nor Dislike	Dislike a Little	Dislike Very Much
WATCHING TV	Not Tried	Like Very Much	Like a Little	Neither Like Nor Dislike	Dislike a Little	Dislike Very Much
PLAYING BALL (Tennis, golf, baseball, football, basketball, etc.)	Not Tried	Like Very Much	Like a Little	Neither Like Nor Dislike	Dislike a Little	Dislike Very Much
READING		Like Very Much	Like a Little	Neither Like Nor Dislike	Dislike a Little	Dislike Very Much
HIKING	Not Tried	Like Very Much	Like a Little	Neither Like Nor Dislike	Dislike a Little	Dislike Very Much
SEEING A MOVIE OR PLAY	Not Tried	Like Very Much	Like a Little	Neither Like Nor Dislike	Dislike a Little	Dislike Very Much

Name:_____

WORKING (paper route, housework, etc.)	Not Tried	Like Very Much	Like a Little	Neither Like Nor Dislike	Dislike a Little	Dislike Very Much
MAKING MODELS	Not Tried	Like Very Much	Like a Little	Neither Like Nor Dislike	Dislike a Little	Dislike Very Much
SWIMMING	Not Tried	Like Very Much	Like a Little	Neither Like Nor Dislike	Dislike a Little	Dislike Very Much
SUNBATHING	Not Tried	Like Very Much	Like a Little	Neither Like Nor Dislike	Dislike a Little	Dislike Very Much
PLAYING CARDS OR OTHER GAMES	Not Tried	Like Very Much	Like a Little	Neither Like Nor Dislike	Dislike a Little	Dislike Very Much
COOKING	Not Tried	Like Very Much	Like a Little	Neither Like Nor Dislike	Dislike a Little	Dislike Very Much
BIKE-RIDING	Not Tried	Like Very Much	Like a Little	Neither Like Nor Dislike	Dislike a Little	Dislike Very Much
WATCHING A BALL GAME	Not Tried	Like Very Much	Like a Little	Neither Like Nor Dislike	Dislike a Little	Dislike Very Much
SHOPPING	Not Tried	Like Very Much	Like a Little	Neither Like Nor Dislike	Dislike a Little	Dislike Very Much
SLEEPING		Like Very Much	Like a Little	Neither Like Nor Dislike	Dislike a Little	Dislike Very Much
HORSEBACK RIDING	Not Tried	Like Very Much	Like a Little	Neither Like Nor Dislike	Dislike a Little	Dislike Very Much

Name:_____

SEWING	Not Tried	Like Very Much	Like a Little	Neither Like Nor Dislike	Dislike a Little	Dislike Very Much
FISHING	Not Tried	Like Very Much	Like a Little	Neither Like Nor Dislike	Dislike a Little	Dislike Very Much
RIDING IN A CAR		Like Very Much	Like a Little	Neither Like Nor Dislike	Dislike a Little	Dislike Very Much
BOATING	Not Tried	Like Very Much	Like a Little	Neither Like Nor Dislike	Dislike a Little	Dislike Very Much
DOING HOMEWORK		Like Very Much	Like a Little	Neither Like Nor Dislike	Dislike a Little	Dislike Very Much
BOWLING	Not Tried	Like Very Much	Like a Little	Neither Like Nor Dislike	Dislike a Little	Dislike Very Much
WORKING ON STAMP OR COIN COLLECTION	Not Tried	Like Very Much	Like a Little	Neither Like Nor Dislike	Dislike a Little	Dislike Very Much
PLAYING A MUSICAL INSTRUMENT	Not Tried	Like Very Much	Like a Little	Neither Like Nor Dislike	Dislike a Little	Dislike Very Much
BABY-SITTING	Not Tried	Like Very Much	Like a Little	Neither Like Nor Dislike	Dislike a Little	Dislike Very Much
SKIING	Not Tried	Like Very Much	Like a Little	Neither Like Nor Dislike	Dislike a Little	Dislike Very Much

Name:_____

If any activities that you like or dislike have been left out of the list, please add them in the spaces below and circle them as you did the others.

	Like Very Much	Like a Little	Neither Like Nor Dislike	Dislike a Little	Dislike Very Much
	Like Very Much	Like a Little	Neither Like Nor Dislike	Dislike a Little	Dislike Very Much
	Like Very Much	Like a Little	Neither Like Nor Dislike	Dislike a Little	Dislike Very Much

QUESTIONNAIRE

INSTRUCTIONS

Each year you are being measured. On this questionnaire we want to find out what type of figure you would like to have and your attitudes about methods of dieting and exercise.

Name_____ Grade_____
           (print)

Address_____

6. Sex (check one)

   □ Male
   1

   □ Female
   0

7–9. In the boxes below write in your estimate of your *present* height:

   7   8 9
   □ Feet   □ Inches

10–12. Now, write in how tall you would *like to be* at your age:

   10   11 12
   □ Feet   □ Inches

13–15. In these boxes estimate your *present weight*:

   13 14 15
   □ Pounds

16–18. Now, write in how much you would *like to weigh* at your present age:

   16 17 18
   □ Pounds

19. How concerned are you about your weight? (check one)

   □ Extremely concerned
   1

   □ Fairly strongly concerned
   2

   □ Only mildly concerned
   3

   □ Not concerned at all
   4

   □ One   UNDERWEIGHT
   5

   □ Two
   6

   □ Three
   7

(leave blank)

20. In general, do you think that you are now (check one) :

☐ Quite a bit too thin
1

☐ A little bit too thin
2

☐ About right
3

☐ A little bit too fat
4

☐ Quite a lot too fat?
5

INSTRUCTIONS

For your present height, would you like to have different proportions?

| Only one check on each line |

	SMALLER	NO CHANGE	LARGER	
21.	☐ 1	☐ 2	☐ 3	Shoulders
22.	☐ 1	☐ 2	☐ 3	Chest (above the bust line)
23.	☐ 1	☐ 2	☐ 3	Waist
24.	☐ 1	☐ 2	☐ 3	Around the hips
25.	☐ 1	☐ 2	☐ 3	Thighs
26.	☐ 1	☐ 2	☐ 3	Calves
27.	☐ 1	☐ 2	☐ 3	Ankles
28.	☐ 1	☐ 2	☐ 3	Biceps
29.	☐ 1	☐ 2	☐ 3	Forearms
30.	☐ 1	☐ 2	☐ 3	Wrists

31. Which one of these places on your body do you think is the farthest from what you would like? (check one)

☐ Shoulders
0

☐ Chest (above the bust line)
1

☐ Waist
2

☐ Around the hips
3

☐ Thighs
4

☐ Calves
5

☐ Ankles
6

☐ Biceps
7

☐ Forearms
8

☐ Wrists
9

EXERCISE

INSTRUCTIONS

If you had to advise a person such as yourself on a plan to develop a good figure, how high would you rate each of the methods of exercise that are described below?

Very high . . . . "6"
Fairly high . . . . "5"
Medium { . . . . "4"
{ . . . . "3"
Fairly low . . . . "2"
Very low . . . . . "1"

32. Doing certain exercises or calisthenics, such as push-ups or kneebends.

☐ ◀ Number from 1 to 6

33. Doing strenuous work.

☐ ◀ Number from 1 to 6

34. Recreational exercise, such as dancing, going for a walk, fishing, going for a horseback or bike ride, going skiing, hiking, going swimming.

☐ ◀ Number from 1 to 6

35. Walking as much as possible instead of riding, such as to school, to work, to go shopping.

☐ ◀ Number from 1 to 6

36. Competitive sports (where you actually compete against other people), such as on a baseball, football, or basketball team, track, volleyball, tennis.

☐ ◀ Number from 1 to 6

DIET

37. What is your opinion of a high school student's cutting out one meal per day and drinking Metrecal or some other liquid diet product instead, as a method of reducing? (check one)

☐ Strongly favor
4

☐ Favor
3

☐ Disapprove
2

☐ Strongly disapprove
1

38. What is your opinion about expecting a high school student to stop drinking *whole* milk and to drink only *skim* milk instead, for a problem of overweight? (check one)

☐ Strongly favor
4

☐ Favor
3

☐ Disapprove
2

☐ Strongly disapprove
1

39. Rate your degree of willingness to go on a diet in which you eat extra amounts of fruits (check one)

☐ 5 High
☐ 4
☐ 3 } In between ◀ One check in any of the boxes
☐ 2
☐ 1 Low

40. Rate your degree of willingness to go on a diet in which you eat extra amounts of vegetables (check one)

☐ 5 High
☐ 4
☐ 3 } In between ◀ One check in any of the boxes
☐ 2
☐ 1 Low

41. What do you think of high school students' taking a daily vitamin pill? (check one)

☐ Very important
3

☐ Of some value
2

☐ No value at all
1

42. What is your opinion about having a high school student eliminate as much fat (mayonnaise, French fries and other fried foods, butter, bacon, fat meat) from his diet as possible as a means of reducing? (check one)

☐ Strongly favor
4

☐ Favor
3

☐ Disapprove
2

☐ Strongly disapprove
1

43. On this question, assume that you are overweight. We want you to rate how willing you would be to eliminate almost all sweets (candy, pastry, soft drinks, etc.) from your diet, if you were overweight.

☐ 6 Very willing to cut out sweets
☐ 5
☐ 4 } In between ◀ One check in any of the boxes
☐ 3
☐ 2
☐ 1 Not willing to cut out sweets

44. Rate your own interest in *learning more* about methods of developing and keeping a good figure (check one).

☐ "I am very interested."
4

☐ "I am somewhat interested."
3

☐ "I am only slightly interested."
2

☐ "I am not interested at all."
1

45. How strong is your willingness to carry out a program of diet to develop a good figure?

☐ 6 Very willing
☐ 5
☐ 4 } In between ◀ One check in any of the boxes
☐ 3
☐ 2
☐ 1 Not willing

46. How strong is your willingness to carry out a program of exercise to develop a good figure?

☐ 6 Very willing
☐ 5
☐ 4 } In between ◀ One check in any of the boxes
☐ 3
☐ 2
☐ 1 Not willing

CASE HISTORIES

O UR GROUP DATA are not definitive in characterizing lean, average, or obese groups because of the wide individual variations within each group. This prompted us to select a few subjects of different types and describe them as individuals. We
hope that these case histories will give our readers a clearer
understanding of the great variety of individuals represented in
our mean values. (The amount of fat or overweight of parents
was obtained as described in Chapter 3.)

Lean Girls

Susan G.

Susan was a tall, pretty, Caucasian girl. She was classified as
lean in the ninth through twelfth grades. She increased five centimeters in height during this time, so that she was growing more
rapidly than the average girl who increased only two centimeters.

She had a low caloric diet of about 1,500 calories a day. Her
intake of calcium, iron, and vitamin A were all below two-thirds
of the Recommended Allowances. However, her intake of ascorbic acid was more than twice the Recommended Allowance because she drank large quantities of orange juice with her meals.

Susan had a very regular pattern of eating, seldom missing
either breakfast or lunch and never missing dinner. She snacked
infrequently. In the ninth grade she reported that dinner was her
favorite meal because "I like salad." In the eleventh grade she
chose breakfast as her favorite and did not state why.

Her total activity score was below the average for the girls as
was the time she spent in moderate and strenuous activity; but
she classified herself as "active." Susan seldom participated in

recreational sports; though she did spend some time almost every day in helping around the house. Her interviewers described her as a "tall, thin, intense-looking girl with large blue eyes. She's quick-moving and always seems in a hurry. She's intelligent and kept a good, if short and concise, record. She never had much to say, but was cooperative and polite." Another said she was a "tall, slender, pretty girl. She seems to be quick-moving and energetic, maybe a little high-strung." So perhaps her activity score was not a true reflection of her actual energy expenditure. On the other hand, it may have been, since she was tall, large-framed, and growing fairly rapidly on a rather low caloric intake.

Susan gave the impression of good health: She was absent from school only once in three years. She made good grades in school, averaged about one and a half hours per day of homework during the school year, and about an hour during the summer when she attended summer school. She usually spent less than an hour a day watching television.

In the ninth grade, Susan classified herself as a little bit too thin. About her food, she said, "I am trying to cut down on fattening foods such as starches and sweets. I would like to stay this way because I feel that within the next few years I will gain weight very rapidly." By the twelfth grade she was extremely concerned about her weight and thought she was a little bit too fat.

This lean girl had a lean mother whom we were able to measure. However, her father was more than 10 percent overweight. Her low caloric consumption, apparently by her own plan and choice, was probably a result of her concern about becoming obese.

Susan's leanness was probably a result of a low caloric consumption in combination with a tall frame and rapid growth. Because she was fairly inactive her activity level perhaps did not contribute much to her caloric expenditure.

Joan K.

This lean Negro girl was growing rapidly from the ninth to the twelfth grades. Joan gained eight centimeters in height during this period, six centimeters more than the average. She was shorter than average in the ninth grade and taller than average in the twelfth grade. She was a late maturer since she did not start to menstruate until age fifteen.

She was a regular eater, missing few meals and not snacking very often. Her diet was fairly good with only calcium below two-thirds of the Recommended Allowance. Her caloric intake was moderate although above the average for the girls, being 2,400 calories per day. In both ninth and eleventh grades, the noon meal was Joan's favorite because she could select her own food at that time. She believed that her own diet was good, and she seemed to have a fairly good knowledge of nutrition. She also indicated that she was trying to "eat a lot and eat fattening foods" to gain weight.

Joan classified herself as average in activity level in the ninth grade and inactive in the twelfth grade. However, her activity score from her record was higher than average for the girls, and she spent more time in strenuous activity than did the average girl. She seemed to have a pleasant social life and impressed her interviewers as friendly and cooperative. She seemed to have a great deal of responsibility at home as she spent much of her time doing housework. She also worked in a cafeteria during her lunch hours while she was in school.

Throughout the study she indicated a concern about her thinness. She seemed to have a realistic opinion of her own size and shape.

Joan was not a scholar as she got poor grades in school, in spite of not being absent very often. Since she reported doing very little homework, she was perhaps not motivated to a high level of scholarship.

Perhaps her rapid growth and higher-than-average level of activity prevented Joan from increasing in fat even though she consumed a higher-than-average level of calories.

Somewhat Lean Girl

Alice S.

Alice was a bouncy, energetic, Caucasian girl. She was somewhat lean and taller than average although not growing very quickly. She increased an average amount in height throughout the study.

Alice seemed to be inconsistent about almost everything. She classified herself as "very inactive" in the ninth grade and "very active" in the twelfth grade. Yet her activity score was consistently above the average for the girls. In the ninth grade she felt that she was "about right" as far as her figure was concerned; nevertheless, she was trying to diet. In the twelfth grade she thought she was a little bit too fat and was fairly concerned about it.

Her pattern of eating, including many snacks, was irregular. This was probably because she usually prepared her own meals. Alice frequently ate breakfast and lunch standing up. In spite of this irregularity, she had a fairly good intake of nutrients except for calcium. Her caloric intake (2,200 calories) was higher than the average for the girls but below the Recommended Allowance. She reported on the ninth-grade questionnaire that dinner was her favorite meal "because there were several varieties of food to eat, and you can have people over and make it into a party." In the eleventh grade she responded to the same question by: "I don't have a favorite meal—they are all the same to me."

Her questionnaire responses indicated that she had little knowledge of the foods that should be eaten every day for health. Yet she was quite positive that teenagers in general had good diets.

Alice showed signs of increasing emotional maturity during the study. Her grades steadily improved from a "C" average in the tenth grade to above a "B" average in twelfth grade. Her school attendance also improved from nine absences in both the tenth and eleventh grades to five in the twelfth grade. Her activity records indicated a great deal of aimless walking around during the first week, with increasing purposeful activity indicated with each succeeding week's record. For example, the second week she participated in church group activities and the third and fourth weeks she had part-time work.

Alice was well coordinated as well as active. She received "A's" or "B's" in physical education and was above average or average in physical performance test scores. She spent more time walking than most of the other girls each of the four weeks that she recorded her activity.

Her mother worked. She was more than 20 percent overweight. Since there was no information available about her father, we assumed that he was not in the home. Also, the lack of meal planning that was evident might indicate this.

We see Alice as a girl who has a fairly good diet and a fairly high level of physical activity. She is also on the lean side of average, all of this happening by accident, so to speak, as there seems to be little regularity or planning in her life.

Average Girl

Debbie L.

This energetic, friendly, attractive Caucasian girl was classified as average in amount of fat and stature. Her height remained the same from the ninth to the twelfth grades.

Debbie was a very good student and had better than average physical performance scores.

She had a fairly regular eating pattern; she always ate breakfast and nearly always ate dinner. However, she missed lunch often and snacked frequently. Her diet was very good. All nutrients were above the Recommended Allowances with the exception of iron, which was above two-thirds of the amount recommended. Her caloric intake was above average for all the girls and above the Recommended Allowances, averaging 2,700 calories.

Her score for recorded activities was above average. She spent more time in moderate and strenuous activities and less time sleeping than did the average girl. She spent more time walking than most of the girls and frequently reported running up and down stairs. In each of the interviewer's notes there was some comment about how active she was, such as "seemed peppy, moved quickly," "She has a lot of pep and moves quickly at all times," or "She is a good swimmer and very *active*." She classified herself as "very active" in the ninth grade and "active" in the twelfth grade.

In spite of her superiority in grades, diet, figure, coordination, and personality, Debbie seemed somewhat dissatisfied with herself. She showed a moderate concern about being a bit fatter than she wanted to be. She graded the healthfulness of her diet as only fair, and she thought she should eat more vegetables, less fat, and fewer desserts. She thought that teenagers did not eat the right foods "because we eat too many sweets and don't eat very nourishing snacks. Quite a few of us skip breakfast."

Although she reported counting calories in the twelfth grade, Debbie indicated in both ninth and twelfth grades that she thought the reason a person was fat was because he did not exercise enough.

We see Debbie as an active girl who was not growing. She was maintaining an average amount of body fat on a higher than average caloric consumption. Her mother was obese. She had in excess of 30 percent body weight as fat and was classified as between 10 and 20 percent overweight. Her father had an average amount of body fat and was not overweight. It would be interesting to see if Debbie continues to maintain her good figure, high activity level, and high caloric intake in adulthood.

Dorothy W.

Dorothy was a very attractive, sociable, tall Negro girl who was classified as average in amount of body fat. She had a large frame and increased an average amount in stature from the ninth to the twelfth grades.

She had a regular eating pattern, seldom missing meals. She consumed only a moderate number of snacks. Her average daily caloric intake was high (2,750 calories) compared to the Recommended Allowance and the other girls in the study. Her overall diet was fairly good, being below two thirds of the Recommended Allowance in only one nutrient, ascorbic acid. One interviewer commented: "Her diet is lacking in fruits and is very high in carbohydrate."

Dorothy was well coordinated, having above average scores in physical performance tests. In spite of this, she showed no interest in athletics. Her activity was mainly light housework, meal preparation, a little walking, physical education in school and occasionally, during the time she was in school, running between classes. She spent a great deal of time watching television, talking on the phone, and sitting and talking with friends. This sociability was remarked by interviewers in the comments: "lovely personality," "pleasing personality," "friendly." Her activity score was below average as was the amount of time she spent in moderate or strenuous activity; but she classified herself as "active."

Even though Dorothy was very attractive and had a "just right" figure, she was mildly concerned about her weight in the tenth grade, and by the twelfth grade she was extremely concerned about being "quite a lot too fat." She also reported that she was doing something about her concern by "not eating many starches, no sweets, lots of fruit, no lunch." However, the food record that she kept in the twelfth grade did not indicate any adherence to this plan.

Dorothy was absent from school rarely in the tenth and eleventh grades, but had ten excused absences and one unexcused absence in the twelfth grade. Her grades were average. She did not seem highly motivated to get good grades as she rarely reported doing any homework.

We have the overall impression of a pretty, pleasant girl with an attractive figure. Although she had a fairly high-calorie diet and was relatively inactive and not growing rapidly, she showed no tendency to become obese. Her father was not overweight, but her mother was more than 10 percent overweight.

It is difficult to explain Dorothy. Possibly her large frame might account for the high-calorie, low-activity pattern existing without obesity. Or, we might speculate since we did not have this information, that her basic metabolic rate was higher than normal.

Somewhat Obese Girl

Norma J.

Norma was a shy, blonde girl, classified as "somewhat obese." From the ninth to the twelfth grade, she increased three centimeters in height, being shorter than average in the ninth grade and of average height in the twelfth grade.

Norma presented many inconsistencies. She complained to the interviewers about poor health but was seldom absent from school. She had a "C" grade average in the tenth grade, below a "C" average in the eleventh grade, and an "A" average in the twelfth grade. Although she seemed disorganized and emotionally unstable, she had much responsibility. She reported doing a great deal of housework and she had a part-time job, while other girls her age engaged in more frivolous activities.

Although her activity score was above average for the girls, she slept a great deal, averaging about eleven and a half hours of sleep out of every 24 hours. She did not appear to be interested in anything.

Norma had a very poor diet with calcium, iron, and thiamine all below two thirds of the Recommended Allowances. Her caloric intake was low, 1,300 calories per day. Her eating pattern was highly irregular. Fairly often she missed breakfasts, lunches, and dinners. She snacked frequently during the summer of 1963, and not frequently at all during subsequent weeks of record-keeping. Although she skipped breakfast often, she selected it as her favorite meal in the ninth grade. Her reason was "After a night's sleep and an early dinner the day before, my energy is almost gone. A good breakfast starts my day with new energy." She graded the healthfulness of her diet as good and did not think it needed improving though we might disagree with her.

She was only moderately concerned about her fatness in ninth and tenth grades, and extremely concerned about it in the twelfth grade. On the twelfth-grade questionnaire, her response to the question of why a person was likely to be fat was "I eat very little, exercise as much as possible, but I know nature didn't intend for me to be fat. There are some people like me with disease which are usually fat."

Her father and his mother were both overweight, but her mother was not.

Norma was somewhat obese throughout her high school years and she did not lose fat on a low-calorie diet. Although her activity score was above average, her hours of sleep seemed almost excessive, and the time she spent in strenuous activity was below average. Her higher than average overall score might be misleading since she was observed to move slowly and behave lethargically.

Norma seemed to have emotional problems and may have

eaten more when not keeping records. At any rate, her failure to lose weight on such a low caloric intake with moderate activity seems puzzling.

Obese Girl Changing to Somewhat Obese

Anne B.

Pretty, short Anne was classified as obese in the ninth grade and somewhat obese in the twelfth grade. She was a Caucasian from the upper socioeconomic group. She was not growing rapidly as she increased an average amount in height. However, she did decrease in amount of body fat.

We were able to measure both her father and mother. Her mother was somewhat lean and her father a little obese. Neither parent however, was classified as overweight.

Anne had a very regular eating pattern: she missed few meals and seldom snacked. Her eating habits seemed to be family-centered with a slight tendency toward food "faddism." She frequently drank water with honey and vinegar in it for breakfast.

Her caloric intake was quite low as was her intake of many nutrients. Calcium, iron, thiamine, and riboflavin were all below two-thirds of the Recommended Allowances. Her low caloric intake appeared to be planned because she drank skim milk and rarely had a starchy vegetable with dinner. In both the ninth and twelfth grades she considered her own diet to be excellent.

Her activity score was below the average for the girls and so was the time she spent in strenuous activity. However, the amount of time she spent in moderate activity was above average, and she classified herself as "active" in both the ninth and twelfth grades.

Her activity records showed that she spent almost no time getting from place to place on foot. She did participate in some active sports though not with any regularity.

She got better than average grades and was absent from school occasionally in the tenth and eleventh grades and frequently in the twelfth grade. Her physical performance scores were below average, but she got "A's" and "B's" in physical education.

She moved fairly slowly and talked quietly. She seemed quite conscientious and had a nice, friendly personality.

In the ninth grade, Anne indicated little concern about her weight and thought she was "about right." In the tenth grade, she was fairly strongly concerned about being "a little bit too fat." However, by the time she was in the twelfth grade, she said she was fairly strongly concerned about being "quite a lot too fat."

She indicated in the ninth grade that she was not on a diet, and in the twelfth grade she said she was "cutting out sweets and cutting down my meals." She reacted to the interviewers with comments that indicated a concern about her diet. She said several times when she had recorded eating ice cream that she should not have eaten it.

Anne seemed to have a tendency to obesity. She had a low caloric intake in spite of a regular eating pattern. Although she lost fat during the study, she did not lose weight. This loss of fat was accompanied by an increased concern about and effort to correct her obesity. She probably did not lose weight or much fat on her low-calorie diet because she was not growing very rapidly and because she was inactive.

Obese Girl

Barbara H.

This short, Caucasian girl was quite pretty in spite of being classified as obese throughout her high school years. Barbara was not growing very fast, increasing only one centimeter in stature from the ninth to the twelfth grade, which was less than the average increase.

Barbara seemed shy, unhappy, and nervous. She seemed to have little social life. She did much of the housework at home. She also spent a great deal of time watching television. For the first week of keeping records, she averaged five hours per day of televiewing, the second week, three hours per day, the third week, four hours per day, and the fourth week, two hours per day. In spite of this, she had a total activity score that was higher than average because she spent more than the average amount of time in moderate and strenuous activity. She participated in recreational sports, including tennis, basketball, badminton, and volleyball, in addition to taking physical education in school. However, we have serious doubts as to just how strenuously Barbara participated in the sports reported because she appeared slow moving, lethargic, and not enthusiastic about anything. She classified herself as average in amount of physical activity in ninth and twelfth grades. Her physical performance scores showed her to be above average in running and ball throwing and below average in sit-ups and the standing broad jump.

Barbara's eating pattern was very irregular; she missed breakfasts, lunches, and dinners. She missed lunch more often than the other meals and seldom snacked. Her diet was very poor: below two thirds of the Recommended Allowances in all nutrients except protein and niacin which were both below Recommended Allowances. Her average caloric intake was extremely low, only 1,150 calories per day.

She had poor grades in school although she was rarely absent.

Her mother had a normal amount of body fat as measured, and there was no information available on her father.

There seems to be no explanation of how Barbara could remain obese on such a low caloric intake and high level of activity as indicated on her records. Since she was highly aware of and concerned about her obesity, she might have actually eaten less and exercised more during the weeks that she kept records, and reverted to a different type of behavior the rest of the year when she did not need to write down what she ate and did. Unless she had a very low basal, or the diary records she kept on food and activity did not reflect her overall pattern of behavior, her case is puzzling.

Somewhat Lean Boy

Jim W.

Jim was a small, neat, quick-moving Negro boy, classified as somewhat lean. He was in the first quintile for height in both the ninth and twelfth grades and was growing quite rapidly for he increased almost twenty centimeters in height during this time.

Jim's caloric intake was above average at 3,000 calories a day, but it was below the Recommended Allowances. His overall diet was fairly good with ascorbic acid being the only nutrient below two thirds of the Recommended Allowances. His pattern of eating was quite irregular. He missed some breakfasts, many lunches, and some dinners. He had his meals at different times from day to day and tended to snack frequently. He seemed to be responsible for his own meal preparation and food choices. He seemed to make fairly good selections, although they were not the traditional foods for the occasion. He cooked himself two hamburgers one morning for breakfast, and several evenings he prepared bacon and eggs or sausage and eggs for an evening meal. Sometimes this was as late as 9:30 P.M. He often prepared hot chocolate for himself, made from evaporated milk. He selected the noon meal as his favorite for reasons of hunger.

Jim had an activity score which was considerably above the average, as was the time he spent in both moderate and strenuous activity. He classified himself as "very active" in the ninth grade and "active" in the twelfth grade. He participated in active sports, including track events, basketball, baseball, and weight-lifting, outside of his physical education class. He tended not to do many inactive things such as television watching, reading, or homework. He was very proud of his well-trained dog, which he brought with him to the interviews on several occasions.

He had higher-than-average school grades but was taking shop courses. He had few absences. His physical performance scores were above average with the exception of sit-ups.

Jim's father and his father's mother were not overweight. There was no information on his mother. In fact, we got the impression that his mother was not in the home. He reported ironing his own clothes and, as already mentioned, seemed to do much of his own meal preparation. In the ninth grade, he listed his father as the expert on good-tasting foods.

He seemed aware of being small but not too concerned about it until he got into the twelfth grade.

Jim probably remained somewhat lean on a higher than average caloric intake because of rapid growth and a high level of physical activity.

Average Boy Changing to Somewhat Lean

Dave D.

"No one could eat as much as this very active Caucasian boy reported eating" was our first outstanding impression of Dave. However, each interviewer questioned him closely about his food intake, particularly quantities, and believed that his record was accurate and did reflect his actual food intake.

He had a fairly regular eating pattern: He skipped lunch occasionally and almost never snacked.

Dave had an average intake of 5,800 calories per day. His intake of all nutrients was well above the Recommended Allowances. He graded the healthfulness of his own diet as "good" rather than "excellent" and said that the only improvement it needed was to include more fruits. (His average intake of ascorbic acid was 430 milligrams per day!)

His favorite meal in both the ninth and eleventh grades was dinner, because "it's the biggest and hot."

This boy was average in height in the ninth grade. He grew ten centimeters to become only slightly above average in the twelfth grade. He was classified as average in amount of body fat in the ninth grade and somewhat lean in the twelfth grade. During this time, he increased about six kilograms in total body weight but increased nearly nine kilograms in lean body weight.

Dave's questionnaire responses indicated that he was satisfied with his own amount of fat and weight but had a typical teenage boy's desire for larger biceps. We were able to measure his mother, and she was quite lean. His father was not overweight.

His total activity score was the highest of all the boys who kept four weeks of records. In spite of this, he classified himself as "active" rather than "very active" in both ninth and twelfth grades.

His activity records indicated that he was a real "go-getter." He did not seem to have time for all the things he did. Dave had jobs all four weeks of the record-keeping. They amounted to at least half-time work for the last three weeks of record-keeping. He also had time to participate in active sports in addition to his physical education classes. He spent almost no time watching television and less time than any other boy in sitting-down types of activity. In the twelfth grade, he checked six "sitting-down" types of activities as disliked very much. These included watching television, listening to radio or records, playing cards, and working on stamp or coin collection.

In spite of the fact that when school was in session he spent from two to two and a half hours a day at homework, he had only average grades. He had a moderate number of absences from school, all of them excused.

He seemed to be quite intense in his attitude toward life. He sat on the edge of his chair during interviews ready to race off as soon as the job was done. One interviewer said of him that he was the type of boy who "would jump over a fence rather than open the gate." He was observed to run up two flights of stairs on several occasions rather than to take the time to wait for the elevator. Just reading over his activity record left one feeling breathless. At one time he reported "loafing" during which time he was walking around.

The picture we see of Dave is that of an average-sized, fast-growing and almost hyperactive individual, who did not get fat on a high caloric diet simply because of a high energy output.

Somewhat Lean Boy Changing to Lean

Frank S.

Frank was a tall, blond, Caucasian boy, classified as somewhat lean in the ninth grade and lean in the tenth through the twelfth grades. His growth rate was average as he gained nine centimeters in height. Both his parents were measured. His father had about an average amount of body fat, while his mother was leaner than average.

Frank had a very regular, home-centered pattern of eating. Although his caloric intake was below Recommended Allowances at 3,300 calories per day, it was above the average of the boys in the study. His intake of all nutrients was either above the Recommended Allowances or close to these levels.

Even though his activity score was below average, he classified himself as "very active" in both the ninth and twelfth grades. This might be because, according to his activity records, he was quite busy. He seemed to have many and varied interests and pursuits. These included piano practice, spectator sports, indoor golf practice, and homework. In other words, he did many things, but the things he did were not very active. He spent much time doing homework when school was in session and had very good grades. He was absent from school only once in three years. In spite of his apparent health, his physical performance scores tended to be average or below.

Frank seemed to be very well adjusted emotionally. He was handsome, charming, and mature except for a refreshingly childlike curiosity about everything. He consistently expressed only mild concern about being a "little bit too thin," throughout the study.

In interviews with him, we got the impression of a happy family life.

In both the ninth and eleventh grades, Frank selected the evening meal as his favorite. Rather typical of the stereotype of the teenagers, his reasons were: "With lunch and breakfast you have a basic or crude choice but with dinner also comes dessert" in the ninth grade, and "It happens to have the best variety and also the servings are bigger" in the eleventh grade. In both grades he indicated that his mother was the person who had "the best idea about good-tasting foods."

Frank was an intelligent, conscientious, pleasant boy who became leaner during his high school years on a caloric consumption that was higher than average. Although not as active as the average boy, he may have needed the higher caloric intake to support his growth and tall frame.

Average Boy Changing to Obese

Jack J.

Jack was a tall, red-haired, slow-moving Caucasian boy who was average in amount of body fat in the ninth, tenth, and eleventh grades and obese in the twelfth. Though tall in the ninth grade, he was still growing as he increased seven centimeters in height between the ninth and eleventh grades. His increase in fat occurred between eleventh and twelfth grades. He appeared to put on fat as soon as he stopped growing.

Unfortunately, we obtained only three weeks of diet and activity records from Jack. We were unable to get him to complete the fourth weeks' diary after he had become obese. Therefore, unlike the other subjects, our comments about him are based on only three records.

His pattern of eating was quite regular. He never missed breakfast and seldom missed lunch or dinner. Although he had very few snacks, he was a heavy eater, averaging nearly 3,800 calories a day. His diet was good. It was close to or above the Recommended Allowances in all nutrients. Jack apparently was aware of this as he graded his own diet as "excellent." In both ninth and eleventh grades he preferred the evening meal. In the ninth grade his reason was "I find I can eat more delicious things." In the eleventh grade he gave as a reason, "It's always hot with lots of good food." In both the ninth and twelfth grades he indicated that cooking was an activity that he liked very much. We certainly get the picture of a "food enthusiast" from these questionnaire responses.

Jack's activity score was below average as was the time he spent in moderate and strenuous activity, but he classified himself as "active."

In the tenth grade Jack was fairly strongly concerned about his weight. However, he thought at the time that he was about right in amount of fatness. In the twelfth grade, after he had become obese, he was only mildly concerned about being a "little bit" too fat. At this time he disapproved the use of liquid formula diets and skim milk and cutting out fats from the diet as weight control measures. In the tenth grade, however, he had approved the use of skim milk and cutting out fats from the diet.

His interviewers commented twice on his personality as being pleasant and his having many interests.

His school grades were below average and so were most of his physical performance scores.

His mother and father were both measured. His mother was obese and his father was normal in amount of body fat.

We see Jack as a large boy who was accustomed to a high caloric consumption and fairly low activity level during a period of rapid growth. He seemed to enjoy food and so, no doubt, continued to eat well after he had stopped growing "up" and started to grow "out."

Obese Boys Changing to Somewhat Obese

Kenneth W.

Kenneth was a tall, slow-moving, slow-talking Negro boy who lost weight (and fat) during the study. He seemed both physically and emotionally mature at our first contact with him. He was obese in the ninth grade and somewhat obese in the twelfth grade. He grew only two centimeters in height and lost 13 kilograms of weight.

Kenneth had a highly irregular pattern of eating. He skipped all meals frequently and snacked often. The meals he did eat were frequently unstructured. His caloric intake was quite low, averaging 1,750 calories. Most nutrients fell below the two-thirds level of Recommended Allowance. There seemed to be no provision or plan for meals in his home.

In both ninth and eleventh grades, Kenneth selected dinner as his favorite meal "because that is the only meal I eat." His diet records seem consistent with this as well as interviewers' notes:

"Big, slow-moving, slow-talking boy. Nice looking and neat. Likeable, polite and friendly. I think he kept an accurate record. I was surprised at how little he ate because of his big frame. He said he wasn't 'hungry' until the afternoon. He doesn't exert himself physically or mentally. He gave up playing the organ after the tenth grade because he said it was too much trouble." This lack of exertion was illustrated by poor grades in school and very low scores in his physical performance tests.

Most of his time was spent in watching television and working in a grocery store. His first week of recorded activities included an average of eight hours a day watching television. Kenneth averaged about ten hours of sleep a night for all four weeks of records. His activity score was below the average of the boys although he classified himself as "average" in the ninth grade and "inactive" in the twelfth grade.

Kenneth appeared to be a tall, fat boy who, while very inactive, did lose weight because of a low caloric consumption. The weight loss seemed to be the result of meal skipping rather than of a deliberate plan or effort.

Bob L.

Bob was a tall, dignified, Negro boy, classified as obese in the tenth grade, and somewhat obese in the twelfth grade. He was not in the study group when he was in the ninth grade. He seemed emotionally mature; but he was still growing physically, as he increased almost nine centimeters in height during the study. At the same time, his amount of body fat was decreasing while he gained slightly in total body weight.

Both of Bob's parents were overweight; his mother was more than 20 percent overweight. Perhaps there was a familial tendency to obesity.

There seemed to be very little structure or organization evident in the family arrangements. Bob missed many meals and had very irregular eating habits. He often prepared his own meals. He was not a frequent snacker. One evening, for instance, Bob consumed five peanut butter and jelly sandwiches and one and one-fourth cups of milk. This was between 5:00 P.M. and 8:00 P.M. while he was lying in bed reading. His other food for that day was lunch which consisted of three bologna and salami sandwiches. In the eleventh grade, he selected lunch as his favorite meal because "I can eat what I want." However, he skipped lunch quite often.

His questionnaire answers indicated that he had a good knowledge of nutrition despite his poor diet. His caloric intake averaged less than 1,800 calories per day, and his intake of all nutrients except riboflavin and niacin was below two-thirds of the Recommended Allowances.

His total score for recorded activities was below average. Bob did not seem to have many interests that were conducive to a high level of activity. He spent from three to four hours a day lying in bed either reading or watching television. On each of two days he spent eight hours watching television (from right after school until late in the evening). During the fourth week of activity record-keeping, when he was a senior, he worked in a grocery store on Saturday and after school.

Although obese with some improvement to the somewhat obese category, Bob was not concerned at all about his weight and was not doing anything about it.

Bob's physical performance scores were below average except for sit-ups in the twelfth grade. His school performance as measured by grade point average and absences was improving from the tenth to the twelfth grade.

This large, rapidly-growing boy appeared to get along on a low caloric intake by being extremely inactive. He lost some fat as well, not by design, but by lack of attention to his food intake.

Somewhat Obese Boy Changing to Obese

Ray B.

Ray did not participate in our study in the ninth grade. He was a pleasant, neat, well-dressed Caucasian boy in the middle socioeconomic class. His height was average, and he was somewhat obese in the tenth grade and obese in the twelfth grade. He was not growing very rapidly, as he increased only five centimeters in height between the tenth and twelfth grades.

His mother was measured and found to have less than the average amount of body fat. Neither of his parents was overweight.

Ray had a regular pattern of eating, missed few meals and snacked frequently. He tended to eat a large amount of bread at mealtime, and often his snacks were high-carbohydrate foods such as cake, candy, soft drinks and ice cream. So, even though he drank skim milk, his caloric intake at 3,000 calories per day was above average for the boys. His intake of nutrients was above two thirds of the Recommended Allowance levels. His records and conversations indicated that his meals were planned and prepared by his mother. He seemed to enjoy food. He said he liked all meals equally well and checked cooking as a well-liked activity.

His activity score was above average as was the time he spent in moderate and strenuous activity. He realistically classified himself as "very active." In addition to taking physical education in school, he seemed to spend much of his time participating in active sports and seemed to walk more than the average boy. He watched television on the average more than two hours a day.

He was only mildly concerned about his weight in the tenth grade and became fairly strongly concerned in the twelfth grade. At both times he thought he was a little bit too fat. He reported that he was "eating a little less and drinking skim milk" to control his weight.

He had steadily improving grades from the tenth to the twelfth grades, and was rarely absent from school. His physical performance scores tended to be below average, in spite of his interest and active participation in sports.

Ray seemed busy and active; his main interests seemed to be watching television and playing at active games with his friends. He was growing and becoming more obese on a higher-than-average caloric intake. Ray is another somewhat puzzling case.

Obese Boys

Bill C.

Bill was a very bouncy, happy, self-assured young man, classified as obese each time he was measured. He was taller than the average boy in the ninth grade but average in height in the twelfth grade. He increased only two centimeters in stature from the ninth to the twelfth grade and so was not growing rapidly, compared to the average boy who increased ten centimeters during this period.

Bill was Caucasian and in the upper socioeconomic class. However, he did not have the typical eating patterns of the other teenagers in these classifications, as his eating habits were quite irregular. He missed many breakfasts, but usually ate lunch and dinner. He had an extremely large number of snacks. One of his interviewers called Bill a "peanut popper" since he seemed to be popping peanuts into his mouth constantly. His snacks were often like small meals. He seemed to be one of the few obese subjects we had who demonstrated a "night-eating syndrome" for he consumed most of his calories after noon and snacked frequently in the evening. One evening he had a hearty dinner at seven, orange juice and an egg salad sandwich at eight, milk and candy at nine-thirty, and a large serving of ice cream at ten. Sometimes he ate dinner at late as ten-thirty in the evening. There seemed to be little reason for this except that he had come home from the Y.M.C.A. at eight-thirty in the evening and watched television from then until ten-thirty. His favorite meal was dinner.

He had a higher than average intake of 3,500 calories a day despite the fact that he often drank skim milk. His intake of all nutrients was above the Recommended Allowances. He graded his own diet as good and believed there was no need to improve it.

Bill did very little homework and did not seem very interested in school, but he had better-than-average grades. He had a moderate number of absences from school. His physical performance scores were average in spite of his pronounced obesity.

Bill was interested in sports but did not participate in them actively. In the eleventh and twelfth grades he was not taking physical education. In the eleventh grade he was excused because he was manager of the basketball team, and in the twelfth grade he worked in the equipment room in the gym instead of taking physical education. He also was a good swimmer, but instead of doing much swimming, he had a job as a life guard or swimming instructor.

His activity score was below average as was the amount of time spent in strenuous activity.

In the ninth, tenth, and twelfth grades, Bill reported that he was "quite a lot too fat," and in the tenth grade he indicated some concern about this with less concern mentioned in the twelfth grade. At no time did he indicate that he had any program to lose weight. He also disapproved of cutting out fats and/ or sweets from the diet as a method of weight reduction.

He did not check many activities as well liked but he did

check cooking as a well-liked activity in both the ninth and twelfth grades.

Bill was friendly and cooperative and well liked by all his interviewers, one of whom described him as bursting with good spirits and life. He seemed to have a lot of energy, and he moved quickly and talked loudly.

He was apparently well adjusted, outgoing, had many interests and, while realistic about his fatness, seemed to be content with himself the way he was.

His father and mother were both measured. His mother had an average amount of body fat and was not overweight, while his father was obese as well as overweight.

Bill selected his father as the authority on good-tasting food. Might this suggest that Bill's father was his male ideal and explain the boy's acceptance of his own obesity?

Bill was maintaining his obesity on a high caloric intake with a lower-than-average energy output in the form of activity and growth and seemed happy with the status quo.

Harold S.

This obese Negro boy increased almost 15 centimeters in height during his high school years. At the same time, he gained in weight and amount of body fat. While he was gaining rapidly in height, he remained a shorter-than-average boy throughout his high school years.

Harold did not seem to let his obesity interfere with his social life. He was popular with the other students as illustrated by the fact that he held a high office in his senior class. He had a pleasant, outgoing personality and a wonderful sense of humor.

In spite of his rapid growth and gain in fat, Harold consumed very few calories (1,600 per day for four weeks). His consumption of many nutrients fell below two-thirds of the Recommended Allowances and reflected an overall poor diet, even though his answers on questionnaires indicated a good knowledge of nutrition. His pattern of eating was quite irregular. He skipped both breakfasts and lunches frequently, breakfast more often, although he was not a frequent snacker. He ate dinner every day.

In both ninth and eleventh grades, dinner was Harold's favorite meal; in ninth grade the reason he gave was that "it is the best and biggest meal" while in the eleventh grade the reason was "have time to eat it and enjoy it—can talk over the day."

In ninth grade in checking a list of well-liked activities, he checked cooking and added eating and relaxing to the list. In spite of his low caloric consumption, Harold seemed interested in food.

According to his activity record, he was slightly above average in total activity score. However, he was observed to walk with some difficulty and move very slowly. Perhaps this difficulty in walking accounted for his low scores on physical performance tests. The only test in which his score did not fall below average was sit-ups. This general inability to perform well physically, along with the observation that he moved slowly, may well indicate that although his score for recorded physical activity was slightly above average, he actually was not as active as he seemed to be from his record.

His overall grade point average in school indicated that he was a better-than-average student. He apparently was seldom ill, as he was seldom absent from school.

We have the overall picture of Harold as a short, fat, rapidly growing teenager. He consumed very few calories, which was a result of meal skipping rather than the selection of low-calorie foods. Meals, when eaten, were inclined to be heavy in fats and carbohydrates. In spite of the low caloric intake and rapid growth, Harold continued to gain fat during the time observed. Contributing factors may have been his short stature, inactivity, and heredity. While his father was not overweight, his mother was 10 to 20 percent overweight.

Summary

It would seem from these case studies that the leanness or fatness of some of our subjects could be easily explained, but that the reasons for the body composition of others presented quite a puzzle. Both food intake and energy expenditure are extremely complicated factors to estimate. The relative contributions of many and varied factors to overall energy expenditure have not been clearly and completely assessed. How much energy is required for growth in relation to total basal metabolism? What is the relative contribution to energy expenditure of physical activity in a rapidly growing teenager, be he sedentary or active? How is the role of heredity in the development of obesity mediated by variations in energy balance? How important are the differences in basal metabolic rates, in growth rates, in body size and composition and amount of energy required for the same activity in different individuals in the development of a lean or obese body?

We can conclude from this look at case histories that teenagers vary widely in patterns of eating, food intakes, and patterns of activity. Perhaps we can assume that the other factors contributing to energy balance vary as widely.